WU 18.2
CHU

(OWL)

Ophthalmology

SCH' `ARY

WES⁊ . 7837

Radcliffe Medical Pr

D1147884

Radcliffe Medical Press Ltd
18 Marcham Road
Abingdon
Oxon OX14 1AA
United Kingdom

www.radcliffe-oxford.com
The Radcliffe Medical Press electronic catalogue and online ordering facility.
Direct sales to anywhere in the world.

British Library Cataloguing in Publication Data

A catalogue record for this book is available from The British Library.

ISBN 1 85775 908 7

Typeset by Aarontype Ltd, Easton, Bristol
Printed and bound by TJ International Ltd, Padstow, Cornwall

Preface

This book is designed to help residents, ophthalmologists and optometrists prepare for the MRCOphth, MRCS, FRCS and final optometry examinations respectively. It also serves as a guide to help comprehensive ophthalmologists update and expand their knowledge of ophthalmology. It is a useful aid for continuing medical education.

The content includes updates in recent scientific trials and studies, medical therapeutics and surgical procedures, covering the subspecialities of cornea and external disease, refractive surgery, cataract, glaucoma, orbital disease and oculoplastics, surgical and medical retina, paediatric ophthalmology, neuro-ophthalmology, uveitis, ocular oncology and pathology. To our knowledge, many of the other previously published self-assessment books have been found to be deficient in these aspects.

A *Fact Finder* is provided at the back of the book.

Chung Nen Chua
September 2002

About the authors

Chung Nen Chua
Specialist Registrar
Oxford Eye Hospital
Oxford

Li Wern Voon
Clinical Corneal Fellow
Oxford Eye Hospital and Nuffield Laboratory of Ophthalmology
University of Oxford
Oxford

and

Registrar
The Eye Institute
Department of Ophthalmology
Tan Tock Seng Hospital
Singapore

Siddhartha Goel
Ophthalmologist
Kent County Ophthalmic and Aural Hospital
Maidstone

How to master MCQs

Multiple choice questions (MCQs) are an effective way of assessing the candidate's knowledge and are an important part of the final MRCOphth/MRCS.

Apart from possessing good knowledge of the subject, we suggest the following tips which we hope will help you excel in the examination.

Remember to answer enough questions

The questions featured in the MRCOphth/MRCS/FRCS examinations are similar. Each question has five parts to be answered. Answers may be True, False or Don't know. +1 mark is given for a correct answer and −1 mark for an incorrect one. No marks are given or deducted for an unanswered question. This system of marking is called negative marking.

The fear of making mistakes may lead to answering too few questions. If the pass mark is 50%, and only half of the questions have been answered with confidence, one may score poorly, as a significant number of answered questions may be wrong. It is recommended that candidates attempt two-thirds of the questions. While this implies making guesses for some of the questions, an intelligent guess based on some background knowledge will more often be right than wrong.

Tricks used by the examiners

1 Pay attention to the phrasing of the question. Phrases that contain the words 'never' or 'always' are usually false, whereas phrases with the word 'may be' are usually true. Good MCQs tend to avoid using these words as much as possible. Other examples are words such as 'typical' or 'rarely'. A sentence may be correct in essence, but not when these phrases are used. For example:

Retinoblastoma:

a   is inherited in the majority of cases

b   arises from receptor cells of the retina

c   is associated with deletion of chromosome 13

d   is typically present with pseudohypopyon

e   that involves the optic nerve has poor prognosis.

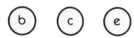

Question **d** illustrates the delicacy of correct phrasing. Pseudohypopyon is a known presentation of retinoblastoma, however, it is not typical.

2   Beware of statements that contain dual information. The first part of the statement may be correct, whereas the second part is incorrect. Mistakes can easily be made if the question is read in a hurry. For example:

In malignant hypertension:

a   intracranial pressure is raised

b   a macular star is caused by the breakdown of the tight junction of the retinal pigment epithelium

c   there is bilateral optic disc swelling with a relative afferent pupillary defect

d   fluorescein angiography may show a dark choroid due to choroidal ischaemia

e   phaeochromocytoma is the most common cause.

In this example, question **c** contains a correct statement in the first part of the question (i.e. malignant hypertension causes bilateral optic disc swelling) but an incorrect statement in the last part (i.e. relative pupillary defect is not a feature of malignant hypertension).

3   Numerical figures in questions are tricky, as they can easily be altered to trick the unwary. It is advisable not to answer these questions unless there is great certainty. For example:

The following are true about primary open-angle glaucoma:

  a   relatives of the affected have an increased incidence of steroid-induced glaucoma

  b   the incidence of a first-degree relative developing the same condition is 1%

  c   dilatation of the pupil always increases the intraocular pressure

  d   abnormality of the trabecular meshwork is often observed during gonioscopy

  e   visual field loss can occur in the presence of normal cup:disc ratio.

When answering this question, one may vaguely remember the value 1% and be pleased to see it in question **b**. The true answer is in fact 10%.

4 Avoid reading too much into the question. For example:

Iritis is a feature of:

    a   systemic lupus erythematosus

    b   psoriatic arthropathy

    c   ulcerative colitis

    d   Behcet's disease

    e   rheumatoid arthritis.

(a)   (b)   (c)   (d)

While rheumatoid arthritis does not cause iritis, some may reason that rheumatoid arthritis-induced scleritis or peripheral corneal melts can give rise to cells in the anterior chamber and hence iritis.

5 Some easy questions may be rendered unanswerable by the use of uncommon vocabulary. For example:

Deuteranomaly:

    a   is caused by an abnormal gene in the X-chromosome

    b   is caused by an abnormality in the green pigment

    c   occurs in about 5% of the European population

    d   is more common than protanomaly

e   is associated with decreased visual acuity.

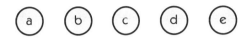

In the question above, deuteranomaly is another term for red–green colour blindness. If one is uncertain of the medical term, it may lead to difficulties in answering the question.

Noting the pearls above will be useful in helping candidates excel in any multiple choice question examination.

1 Vigabatrin:

a is used as the first-line medication in grand mal epilepsy

b increases GABA concentration in the retina

c causes visual field defects in one-third of patients

d is contraindicated in patients with pre-existing visual field defect

e causes narrowing of the retinal arterioles.

2 The following pharmacological tests are useful in differentiating a patient with a fixed dilated pupil:

a 4% cocaine test

b 0.01% pilocarpine

c 1% pilocarpine

d 2.5% phenylephrine

e 0.1% adrenaline.

3 Kayser-Fleischer's ring:

a is pathognomonic of Wilson's disease

b first appears in the superior and inferior Descemet's membrane

c occurs in all patients with hepatic failure due to Wilson's disease

d occurs in all patients with neurologic manifestations of Wilson's disease

e disappears with desferrioxamine treatment.

4 Ocular signs associated with abnormal dentition are seen in:

a congenital syphilis

b Reiger's syndrome

c congenital rubella

d Down's syndrome

e pseudoxanthoma elasticum.

1

Vigabatrin is used in combination with other anti-epileptics in the control of epilepsy. It is not used as a first-line treatment except in West's syndrome. It increases the concentration of GABA in the brain and the retina. It is associated with visual field defects (as many as one-third of patients) but the mechanism is unknown. It should be avoided in patients with pre-existing visual field defect. Ophthalmoscopy appearance in patients taking vigabatrin includes narrowing of the retinal arterioles, wrinkles on the retina surface and optic atrophy in the presence of visual field defects.

2

Cocaine test is used to confirm Horner's syndrome and 2.5% phenylephrine or 0.1% adrenaline are used to localise the site in Horner's syndrome. 0.01% pilocarpine causes constriction of Adie's pupil and 1% pilocarpine will constrict a dilated pupil caused by third nerve palsy but will not constrict a pharmacologically dilated pupil.

3

Kayser-Fleischer's ring is not pathognomonic for Wilson's disease; it can occur in other conditions such as primary biliary cirrhosis. In patients with suspected Wilson's disease, gonioscopy may be required to detect early copper deposition at the periphery of Descemet's membrane in the superior and inferior limbus. It may be absent in patients with hepatic failure due to Wilson's disease but is always present in those with neurologic manifestations. It disappears with D-penicillamine treatment.

4

Congenital syphilis can give rise to Hutchinson's teeth and Reiger's syndrome is associated with under-developed dentition.

Quick fix

- *Drugs that can cause retinal pigment epithelial dysfunction:* (hydroxyl)chloroquine, phenothiazine and desferrioxamine.

- *Drugs that can cause macular oedema:* nicotinic acid, latanoprost and topical adrenaline.

- *Drugs that can cause crystalline retinopathy:* tamoxifen, methoxyflurane and canthaxanthine.

5 Location of lesion for the following abnormal ocular movements are true:

a   WEBINO (wall-eyed bilateral internuclear ophthalmoplegia) – rostral medial longitudinal fasciculus and the third nerve nucleus

b   internuclear ophthalmoplegia – contralateral medial longitudinal fasciculus

c   one and a half syndrome – ipsilateral medial longitudinal fasciculus and ipsilateral sixth nerve nucleus

d   down-gaze palsy – caudal interstitial nucleus of the medial longitudinal fasciculus

e   skew deviation – ipsilateral sixth and third nerve nucleus.

6 Idiopathic polypoidal choroidal vasculopathy (IPCV):

a   occurs mainly in people of African descent

b   drusen are typically absent

c   causes vitreous haemorrhage

d   is best visualised with indocyanine green

e   has a better visual prognosis than age-related macular degeneration.

7 The following are true about pigment dispersion syndrome:

a   peripapillary transillumination is a feature

b   the anterior chamber is deeper than the normal population

c   the iris is inserted more posteriorly into the ciliary body than the normal population

d   exercise or pupil dilatation causes intraocular pressure to rise

e   there is an increased incidence of lattice degeneration.

8 Aberrant regeneration of the oculomotor nerve:

a   presents with retraction of the upper lid on down-gaze

b   presents with miosis on attempted adduction

c   has not been reported in oculomotor palsy caused by diabetes

d   most often occurs after trauma or aneurysm

e   is suggestive of orbital meningioma in the absence of antecedent oculomotor nerve palsy.

5 (a) (c)

Internuclear ophthalmoplegia is caused by a lesion in the ipsilateral medial longitudinal fasciculus, i.e. the same side as the eye that has adduction restriction. Down-gaze palsy is caused by a lesion in the rostral interstitial nucleus of the medial longitudinal fasciculus. The lesion for skew deviation is in the brain stem but the exact location is unknown.

6 (b) (c) (d) (e)

IPCV was first described in people of African descent but it is now being recognised in other races due to increased awareness. The condition typically affects women in the fifth and sixth decade. Haemorrhage is common and it was previously called posterior uveal bleeding syndrome. It is one of the differential diagnoses of age-related macular degeneration (ARMD). Unlike ARMD, it is not associated with drusen. The lesions are made up of dilated choroidal vessels and are best visualised with indocyanine green. IPCV tends to affect the peripapillary region away from the fovea. Therefore, the outcome of treatment is more favourable than ARMD.

7 (b) (c) (d) (e)

Pigment dispersion syndrome is associated with pigmentary glaucoma and the risk factors are myopia and raised intraocular pressure. In this condition, the pigment dispersion is believed to be caused by the rubbing of the iris against the lens. This is caused by concavity of the iris as a result of a more posteriorly inserted iris. Iridotomy is useful in reducing the iris–lens contact and hence the amount of pigment dispersed. Lattice degeneration is increased in pigment dispersion syndrome as most of the sufferers are myopic.

8 (a) (b) (c) (d) (e)

Aberrant regeneration of the oculomotor nerve occurs in a 'surgical' third nerve palsy and not in 'medical' third nerve palsy such as diabetes mellitus or hypertension. Retraction of the upper lid on down-gaze is called pseudo von Graefe's sign and miosis of the pupil on adduction is termed pseudo Argyll-Robertson pupil.

9 True autofluorescence is a feature of:

a optic disc drusen

b macular drusen

c cotton wool spots

d myelinated nerve fibres

e astrocytic hamartoma.

10 With regard to optic neuritis:

a 95% of patients recover their vision to 6/12 or better

b the risk of developing multiple sclerosis is higher in patients with a T2 weighted abnormal MRI scan

c a faster visual recovery occurs with systemic corticosteroids

d final visual outcome is improved with systemic corticosteroids

e the risk of developing multiple sclerosis is reduced in patients treated with corticosteroids.

11 The following are true about the differences between LASIK (laser assisted in-situ keratomileusis) and PRK (photorefractive keratectomy):

a LASIK is technically easier to perform than PRK

b LASIK can be used to treat a higher myopia than PRK

c LASIK causes less pain than PRK

d LASIK is associated with less regression than PRK

e epithelial downgrowth is seen in LASIK but not PRK.

12 In Stickler's syndrome:

a type II collagen is defective

b high myopia of more than 8 diopters is a feature

c bone-spicule pigmentary changes are common in the peripheral retina

d retinal detachment affects about 50% of patients

e epiphyseal dysplasia of the long bones is a feature.

9

Autofluorescence is defined as the emission of fluorescent light from ocular structures in the absence of sodium fluorescein. On the other hand, pseudo-autofluorescence results from reflection of light from light-coloured or white fundal structures such as myelinated nerve fibres, sclera, hard exudates or cotton wool spots.

11

LASIK involves the creation of a partial thickness corneal flap followed by photorefractive surgery. It is technically more difficult than PRK. However, it has the advantages of faster visual rehabilitation with less pain and the ability to treat higher myopia. Epithelial downgrowth can occur under the flap in LASIK, resulting in poor vision.

10

Systemic corticosteroids can speed up the visual recovery of optic neuritis but the final visual outcome does not appear to be affected. It does not prevent the development of multiple sclerosis.

12

Stickler's syndrome is an autosomal dominant condition. The patient has abnormal type II collagen, with high myopia (>8D), perivascular pigmentary changes but no bone-spicule formation. There is empty vitreous and the incidence of retinal detachment is as high as 50%. Orofacial anomalies are common, as are joint changes, especially at the epiphyses of the long bones.

Quick fix

- The Optic Neuritis Treatment Trial (ONTT) showed that high-dose IV corticosteroids followed by oral corticosteroids accelerated visual recovery, but provided no long-term benefit to vision.

- Oral corticosteroids alone did not improve visual outcome and were associated with an increased rate of recurrence of optic neuritis.

- IV followed by oral corticosteroids reduced the rate of development of clinically definite multiple sclerosis during the first 2 years, particularly in patients with white lesions detected on MRI of the brain. This positive effect was no longer evident after 2 years.

13 In a patient with symptomatic right superior oblique palsy, the following surgery may be useful:

a right inferior oblique anterior transposition

b left inferior oblique myectomy

c left inferior rectus recession

d right superior rectus resection

e right superior oblique tuck.

14 Increased pigmentary deposition in the angles is seen in:

a pseudoexfoliation syndrome

b patients on latanoprost treatment

c pigment dispersion syndrome

d laser iridotomy

e oculodermal melanocytosis.

15 The following are true about the structures seen on gonioscopy:

a Sampaolesi's line is anterior to Schwalbe's line

b Scheie's stripe is located within the trabecular meshwork

c the scleral spur is the posterior border of the trabecular meshwork

d Schwalbe's line marks the termination of Descemet's membrane

e the scleral spur defines the anatomical limbus.

16 Regarding Wernicke's encephalopathy:

a vitamin B_1 deficiency is the underlying cause

b occurs in hyperemesis gravidarum

c lesions typically occur in the frontal lobe

d ophthalmoplegia occurs as the result of peripheral cranial nerve palsies

e cerebellar signs are characteristic.

13

A right superior oblique palsy can result in vertical or torsional diplopia. Vertical diplopia may be treated with either ipsilateral inferior oblique myectomy or anterior transposition, contralateral inferior rectus recession or ipsilateral superior oblique tuck (sometimes in combination). Torsional diplopia can be treated with anterior transposition of the superior oblique muscle.

15

Sampaolesi's line is caused by pigment deposition and is found anterior to Schwalbe's line. Scheie's stripe is outside the trabecular meshwork and refers to the area of pigmentation between the lens zonules and the lens capsule. The anterior border of the trabecular meshwork is defined by Schwalbe's line and the scleral spur defines the posterior border. The anatomical limbus is defined by Schwalbe's line.

14

Latanoprost increases melanin production in the melanocytes but does not cause increased pigmentary deposition in the angle.

Quick fix

- Differentiation of unilateral from bilateral fourth nerve palsy is essential for successful surgical management.

- Features of unilateral fourth nerve palsy include: head tilt to the affected side, unilateral hypertropia on lateral gaze, less than 5° of exocyclotorsion.

- Features of bilateral fourth nerve palsy include: chin down posture with eyes looking up, alternating hypertropia on right and left gaze respectively, large exocyclotorsion of more than 10°.

16

Wernicke's encephalopathy is characterised by ophthalmoplegia, mental confusion and gait ataxia. It is caused by vitamin B_1 deficiency and is commonly seen in alcoholics. It also occurs in hyperemesis gravidarum in which the pregnant woman cannot take in food due to recurrent vomiting. The ophthalmoplegia is central in origin. Lesions are found in the motor and vestibular nuclei, paraventricular region of the thalamus, hypothalamus and the cerebellum.

17 The following are true about Leber's hereditary optic neuropathy:

a it causes painless visual loss in young patients

b Uhthoff's phenomenon is a recognised symptom

c affected males do not pass the condition to their offspring

d fluorescein angiography shows leakage of dye at the optic disc

e the amount of recovery can be predicted from the genetic mutation.

18 The following signs are regarded as significant macular oedema in diabetes mellitus:

a microaneurysms within one disc diameter of the fovea

b hard exudate in the fovea

c retinal thickening within 500 μm of the fovea

d retinal thickening of one disc diameter, any part of which is within one disc diameter of the fovea

e flamed haemorrhages within 500 μm of the fovea.

19 The following blood tests are useful for the respective diseases mentioned:

a C-ANCA in Wegener's granulomatosis

b P-ANCA in polyarteritis nodosa

c anticentromere antibody in scleroderma

d anti-SS-B in primary Sjogren's syndrome

e anti-striated muscle antibody in thymoma.

20 The Gram stain of a patient's corneal ulcer reveals Gram-negative rods. The following are possible diagnoses:

a *Pseudomonas aeruginosa*

b *Corynebacterium*

c *Serratia marcescens*

d *Moraxella*

e *Neisseria.*

17

Painless visual loss differentiates Leber's optic neuropathy from optic neuritis. Uhthoff's phenomenon describes decreased vision with exercise or warming of body temperature and is seen in both optic neuritis and Leber's hereditary optic neuropathy, as well as in other optic neuropathies. The condition is caused by abnormalities in the mitochondrial DNA and therefore is not transmitted in sperm. Ophthalmoscopy reveals circumpapillary telangiectatic microangiopathy and swelling of the nerve fibre layer around the disc. However, unlike in patients with swollen disc, leakage of dye is not seen in fluorescein angiography. The type of mutation can predict visual recovery, those with 117788 mutation have poor recovery, whereas those with 14484 mutation have significant visual recovery.

18

Clinically significant macular oedema is defined as:

- retinal thickening within 500 μm of the fovea
- presence of hard exudate with retinal thickening within 500 μm of the fovea
- retinal thickening of one disc diameter and any part of which is within one disc diameter of the fovea.

19

ANCA is present in polyarteritis nodosa and Wegener's granulomatosis. Perinuclear ANCA (P-ANCA) is seen in polyarteritis nodosa whereas cytoplasmic ANCA (C-ANCA) is seen in Wegener's granulomatosis.

20

Corynebacterium is a Gram-positive rod and *Neisseria* is a Gram-negative coccus. *Pseudomonas aeruginosa* is the most common pathogen in contact lens-related corneal ulcer. *Serratia marcescens* is uncommon but can cause rapid and extensive corneal necrosis. *Moraxella* species are opportunistic pathogens and are usually seen in alcoholic or debilitated patients.

Quick fix

- The Diabetes Control and Complications Trial (DCCT) showed that tight glycaemic control in type I diabetes mellitus delayed onset and progression of diabetic retinopathy, neuropathy and nephropathy.

- The United Kingdom Prospective Diabetes Study (UKPDS) showed that tight control of blood glucose and hypertension in type II diabetes mellitus reduces the risk of diabetic eye disease and macrovascular disorders such as stroke and renal disease.

21 In Miller-Fisher's syndrome:

a two-thirds of patients present with diplopia

b the ratio of male to female involvement is about 2 : 1

c the cerebrospinal fluid shows lymphocytosis

d antibody to ganglioside GQ 1b is diagnostic

e chronic cases occur in 50% of patients.

22 With regard to progressive supranuclear palsy:

a it occurs in patients with chronic Parkinson's disease

b the vertical eye movements are affected before the horizontal eye movements

c the downward pursuit movement is usually affected before the upward pursuit movement

d blinking to bright light is reduced

e oral levodopa improves the eye movement in the majority of patients.

23 In infantile esotropia:

a amblyopia occurs in 40% of patients despite early surgery

b early surgical correction restores normal binocular single vision

c asymmetric optokinetic nystagmus occurs with a better nasal-to-temporal movement than temporal-to-nasal movement

d 90% of patients have dissociated vertical deviation

e post-surgical accommodative esotropia is common.

24 The following are true about retinoblastoma:

a a family history is present in less than 10% of the sufferers

b about 40% of all cases of retinoblastoma are heritable

c deletion of 13q14 chromosome is seen in 25% of patients

d systemic malformations are more common in those with bilateral than unilateral retinoblastoma

e secondary cancers are more common in non-heritable than heritable retinoblastoma.

21

Miller-Fisher's syndrome is a variant of Guillain Barre's syndrome. It is characterised by areflexia, external ophthalmoplegia and ataxia. Diplopia is the most common presentation. The cerebrospinal fluid typically shows dissociation of proteins and cells, i.e. the protein is increased but there are minimal cells. Chronic or recurrent cases are uncommon.

22

Progressive supranuclear palsy is a form of parkinsonism, which is different from Parkinson's disease. The vertical eye movement is affected early before the horizontal eye movement. Both the saccades and pursuit movements are abnormal. The blinking reflex is also affected. Unlike Parkinson's disease, it does not respond to levodopa.

23

Infantile esotropia has large angle esotropia. Binocular single vision is usually poor despite early treatment. The temporal-to-nasal movement is usually better than nasal-to-temporal movement on optokinetic testing. Dissociated vertical deviation and inferior oblique overaction are common and have been reported in about 90% of patients. Post-surgical esotropia may be caused by an accommodative component.

24

About 40% of all retinoblastomas are caused by germinal mutation and are therefore heritable. Deletion of 13q14 occurs in about 1% of cases and is associated with systemic malformation. Heritable retinoblastoma is associated with a higher incidence of secondary cancers.

Quick fix

- Genetics of retinoblastoma are as follows: 94% sporadic and 6% familial.
- Patients with bilateral retinoblastoma and some cases of unilateral retinoblastoma may have germline mutation.
- The risk of offspring having the disease is as follows:
  - if one parent has retinoblastoma: 40%
  - if both parents are normal and one sibling has unilateral retinoblastoma: 1%
  - if both parents are normal and one sibling has bilateral retinoblastoma: 6%.

25 In shaken baby syndrome:

a the average age of the patient is about 2 years old

b retinal haemorrhages are essential for the diagnosis

c retinal haemorrhages are useful in determining the time of trauma

d neurological deficits occur in about one-third of patients

e permanent visual loss results from retinal lesions.

26 Risk factors for expulsive suprachoroidal haemorrhage during cataract extraction include:

a high myopia

b history of glaucoma

c shallow anterior chamber

d atherosclerosis

e blue iris.

27 The following are true about the use of pneumatic retinopexy:

a it is contraindicated in patients with glaucoma

b it is not suitable for patients with inferior retinal detachment

c presence of any proliferative vitreoretinopathy is a contraindication

d the retinal breaks should be within one clock hour of each other

e the success rate is higher in pseudophakic compared with phakic patients.

28 The advantages of continuous curvilinear capsulorrhexis over capsulotomy include:

a easier prolapse of the lens nucleus into the anterior chamber

b ensures 'in the bag' intraocular lens implantation

c allows hydrodissection of the lens with minimal risk of extension of tear to the equator

d reduced incidence of post-operative intraocular lens decentration

e reduced incidence of posterior capsule thickening.

25

Retinal haemorrhages are commonly seen in shaken baby syndrome. However, they are not necessary for diagnosis and should not be used to determine the time of trauma. Neurological deficits occur in about one-third of patients. Visual impairment is usually caused by cerebral damage.

26

Expulsive suprachoroidal haemorrhage is rare and has been estimated to occur in about one in every thousand cases of cataract extraction. Risk factors include increased axial length, glaucoma, atherosclerosis and previous expulsive suprachoroidal haemorrhage.

Quick fix

The risk of expulsive haemorrhage during cataract surgery may be reduced by the following measures:

- small incision surgery
- control of intraocular pressure
- control of systemic hypertension.

27

Pneumatic retinopexy involves the use of air to flatten the retina following cryotherapy. It is suitable only for superior retinal detachment and the retinal tears should be within one clock hour of each other. As there is often an increase in intraocular pressure, it is contraindicated in glaucoma. Grade C PVR is a contraindication as the retina is usually rigid in these cases. The success rate is higher in phakic than pseudophakic patients.

28

Capsulorrhexis allows safe hydrodissection and phacoemulsification. It ensures 'in-the-bag' intraocular lens implantation and reduced post-operative decentration. Nucleus prolapse is difficult in capsulorrhexis compared with capsulotomy. Capsulorrhexis does not reduce the incidence of posterior capsule thickening.

29 In involutional ptosis:

a height of the skin crease is increased

b levator function is reduced

c ptosis is decreased on down-gaze

d up-gaze is usually abnormal

e levator resection is the treatment of choice.

30 An increased rate of proliferative vitreoretinopathy is seen in:

a multiple retinal breaks

b pneumatic retinopexy

c scleral buckling

d vitrectomy surgery

e vitreous haemorrhage.

31 The following lens changes are typical of the medical condition mentioned:

a posterior subcapsular cataract in retinitis pigmentosa

b anterior subcapsular cataract in amiodarone user

c posterior lenticonus in Alport's syndrome

d droplet cataract in galactosaemia

e polychromatic cataract in Wilson's disease.

32 In a patient with subluxated lens, the following tests are useful:

a echocardiogram

b serum methionine

c brain MRI

d serum FTA antibodies

e urine thiosulphate.

29

In involutional ptosis, there is dehiscence of the levator aponeurosis resulting in an elevated skin crease. The ptosis is constant in up- or down-gaze. The up-gaze is not affected as in some congenital ptosis. Levator advancement is the treatment of choice.

30

Proliferative vitreoretinopathy is thought to be caused by the release of retinal pigment epithelium onto the retina. The incidence of PVR is increased in large or multiple retinal breaks, cryotherapy, vitreous haemorrhages and vitrectomy surgery. Pneumatic retinopexy and scleral buckling do not increase PVR.

31

Amiodarone can give rise to anterior stellate deposit but is usually visually insignificant. Alport's syndrome is associated with anterior lenticonus. Polychromatic cataract is seen in myotonic dystrophy.

32

Echocardiogram may show enlarged aortic roots or mitral valve prolapse in Marfan's syndrome. High serum methionine is seen in homocystinuria. Syphilis is a known cause of ectopia lentis. Urine thiosulphate is seen in sulphite oxidase deficiency, in which the disulphide bond is disrupted and can cause ectopia lentis.

Quick fix

Drugs that cause vortex keratopathy include:

- amiodarone
- (hydroxyl) chloroquine
- chlorpromazine
- indomethacin
- mepacrine
- tamoxifen.

33 Shallowing of the anterior chamber during phacoemulsification may indicate:

a posterior capsule rupture

b retinal detachment

c suprachoroidal haemorrhage

d inadequate infusion of BSS

e aqueous misdirection syndrome.

34 The following are true about the Endophthalmitis Vitrectomy Study:

a use of vancomycin in the irrigating solution reduces the risk of endophthalmitis

b *Staphylococcus aureus* is the most common pathogen

c systemic corticosteroid is useful

d intravenous antibiotic improves the final visual outcome

e vitrectomy is only useful in patients with light-perception vision.

35 The risk of zonular dehiscence during cataract surgery is increased in the following conditions:

a pseudoexfoliation syndrome

b pigment dispersion syndrome

c aniridia

d Ehler-Danlos syndrome

e albinism.

36 Concerning malignant glaucoma:

a it occurs most commonly after filteration surgery for acute angle-closure glaucoma

b the anterior chamber is typically shallow

c the volume of the vitreous is increased

d the increased pressure is due to anterior displacement of the ciliary body by choroidal effusion

e the pressure can be controlled with a miotic.

33

Shallowing of the anterior chamber can result from inadequate fluid infusion or a rise in vitreous pressure. The latter can result from breath holding, pressure from the speculum, or misdirection of the aqueous or suprachoroidal haemorrhage. Posterior capsule rupture and retinal detachment usually cause deepening of the anterior chamber.

34 ⓔ

The study did not look into the use of vancomycin or systemic corticosteroid in endophthalmitis. The most common pathogen is *S epidermidis*. In the study, intravenous antibiotic did not appear to affect the outcome. Vitrectomy appeared to improve the visual outcome in those with light perception only.

35

The zonules are weakened in patients with pseudoexfoliation syndrome, aniridia and Ehler-Danlos syndrome. Other conditions that can increase zonular dehiscence include high myopia, syphilis, Marfan's syndrome, Weil-Marchesani syndrome, sulphate oxidase deficiency and lysine deficiency.

36 ⓐ ⓑ ⓒ

Malignant glaucoma typically occurs following trabeculectomy in angle-closure glaucoma. The anterior chamber is shallow with raised intraocular pressure. The mechanism is believed to be caused by aqueous misdirection, resulting in expansion of the vitreous, causing forward movement of the lens and the ciliary body. The initial treatment of choice is a cycloplegic which moves the lens backwards and encourages the flow of aqueous anteriorly.

Quick fix

- High intraocular pressure following trabeculectomy can be the result of either angle-closure glaucoma or malignant glaucoma.

- In angle-closure glaucoma, a non-patent iridectomy is the usual cause. In malignant glaucoma, the iridectomy is patent.

- In malignant glaucoma, the initial treatment of choice is medical with mydriatics and intravenous hyperosmotic agents.

37 Uveitis and poliosis are seen in:

a sympathetic ophthalmia

b Vogt-Koyanagi-Harada's syndrome

c AZOOR

d tuberculosis

e sarcoidosis.

38 With regard to acute retinal necrosis:

a the affected eye is usually painless

b the condition is bilateral in one-third of cases

c retinal detachment is an important cause of visual loss

d most patients are immunocompromised

e gancyclovir is the treatment of choice.

39 The following are true about retinal capillary haemangioma:

a it is usually the first manifestation of von Hippel-Lindau's syndrome

b radiological imaging of the abdomen and head should be carried out irrespective of family history

c spontaneous regression is common and close observation is the management of choice

d there is usually a prominent feeding vessel but normal drainage vessel

e a blood test may show thrombocythaemia.

40 An HIV-positive patient was found to have a white lesion on the retina. The following can accurately differentiate a cotton wool spot from CMV retinitis:

a CD4+ count

b presence of vitritis

c visual acuity

d presence of haemorrhage

e enlargement of the lesion.

37

Pigment abnormalities are seen in sympathetic ophthalmia and VKH syndrome, which can also cause uveitis.

38

Acute retinal necrosis usually presents with a painful red eye and panuveitis. It usually affects immunocompetent patients. Herpes viruses, especially herpes simplex and varicella zoster, are often implicated. Visual loss is usually due to optic neuritis and retinal detachment. The treatment of choice is initial intravenous acyclovir followed by an oral course. Gancyclovir is not used due to its toxicity and the need for intravenous administration to be effective.

39

Retinal capillary haemangioma is often the first manifestation of von Hippel-Lindau's syndrome. As the disease may skip a generation(s), a MRI scan of the abdomen and head for potentially lethal tumours such as phaeochromocytoma or cerebellar haemangioblastoma is essential. The lesions have variable progression, and ablation with either cryotherapy or photocoagulation is recommended before the tumour gets too big. Both the feeding and drainage vessels are usually enlarged. Cerebellar haemangioblastoma can give rise to polycythaemia through erythropoietin secretion, and the blood tests show increased red blood cells.

40

Early CMV retinitis can pose a diagnostic dilemma as it may resemble cotton wool spots which are common in HIV patients. Although CMV retinitis is more common in those with CD 4+ counts of fewer than 50 cells per μl, it cannot be used to differentiate the two conditions. Furthermore, early CMV retinitis is asymptomatic and vitritis is minimal. White lesions in HIV patients should be observed over time for any enlargement or development of haemorrhages which are suggestive of CMV retinitis.

41 The following are true about the optokinetic response:

a   it tests the pursuit movement in the direction of the movement of the drum

b   a subject who has a right pursuit problem is likely to have a lesion in the left parietal lobe

c   a subject who has a problem with refixation when the drum is moved to the left is likely to have a lesion in the left frontal lobe

d   a patient with Parinaud's syndrome will develop convergence retraction nystagmus when the drum is rotated vertically

e   in a patient with adduction deficit, the presence of adduction in response to an optokinetic drum indicates a supranuclear lesion.

42 Enlarged superior ophthalmic vein on CT scan is a feature in:

a   carotid cavernous fistula

b   posterior communicating artery aneurysm

c   craniopharyngioma

d   von Hippel-Lindau's syndrome

e   cavernous sinus thrombosis.

43 The following are true about neonatal conjunctivitis:

a   it is defined as conjunctivitis that occurs within 28 days of birth

b   chlamydial conjunctivitis is the most common cause in the UK

c   topical tetracycline is the treatment of choice in chlamydial conjunctivitis of the neonate

d   Thayer-Martin medium is useful in isolating *Neisseria gonorrhoea*

e   topical treatment should be combined with systemic treatment in gonococcal conjunctivitis.

44 In familial exudative vitreoretinopathy:

a   males are more commonly affected than females

b   dragged discs may be present which can be confused with retinopathy of prematurity

c   fluorescein angiography shows failure of vascularisation of the temporal retina

d   exudative retinal detachment is the most common cause of poor vision

e   prophylactic cryotherapy of the peripheral retina is useful in preventing visual loss.

41

Optokinetic response tests the pursuit and saccadic movements. When the drum is rotated to the right, the pursuit movement is mediated by the right parietal lobe and the saccadic movement by the right frontal lobe, i.e. the optokinetic response tests the pursuit and saccadic movement on the side towards which the drum is moving. Parinaud's syndrome causes up-gaze palsy and vertical rotation of the drum will elicit convergence retraction nystagmus. In a patient with a frontal lobe lesion, there may be deviation of his or her eyes to the side of the lesion. However, provided the contralateral frontal lobe is intact, rotating an optokinetic drum away from the side of the frontal lobe will elicit a response.

42

Enlarged superior ophthalmic vein occurs when the drainage of venous blood into the cavernous sinus is impaired. This occurs in carotid cavernous fistula and cavernous sinus thrombosis. The other conditions mentioned do not increase the pressure of the cavernous sinus or impair venous drainage.

43

Chlamydial conjunctivitis is the most common cause of neonatal conjunctivitis. Systemic antibiotics such as erythromycin are indicated due to the high risk of pneumonitis. Thayer-Martin medium contains antibiotic and antifungal agents that will stop the growth of bacteria and fungus but not that of *Neisseria gonorrhoea*. Like chlamydial conjunctivitis, gonococcal conjunctivitis should also be treated with systemic antibiotics.

44

Familial exudative vitreoretinopathy is an autosomal dominant condition. Clinically it may resemble retinopathy of prematurity with failure of vascularisation in the temporal retina leading to fibrovascular changes with dragged macula and disc. However, a history of prematurity is absent. Although exudates are common, retinal detachment is rare. Poor vision usually results from rheumatogenous retinal detachment. The use of cryotherapy or photocoagulation to the avascular retina reduces complications.

45 The following maculopathies typically give rise to severe central visual loss before the age of 40:

a Sorby's macular dystrophy

b Stargardt's macular dystrophy

c Best's disease

d central areolar choroidal dystrophy

e North Carolina macular dystrophy.

46 Corneal blood staining following hyphaema is increased in:

a raised intraocular pressure

b a patient with sickle cell anaemia

c prolonged hyphaema

d Fuch's endothelial dystrophy

e use of topical steroid.

47 Presence of the following condition decreases the risk of proliferative diabetic retinopathy:

a advanced glaucoma

b pseudoxanthoma elasticum

c high myopia

d posterior vitreous detachment

e renal failure.

48 The following are true about corticosteroid-induced ocular hypertension:

a diabetes is a risk factor

b the ocular hypertension is caused by outflow obstruction

c it is related to the strength of the topical steroid used

d the time from taking the steroid to development of ocular hypertension is longer for systemic than for topical steroid

e ocular hypertension which fails to reverse after stopping corticosteroid is more common in myopia.

45

All the conditions mentioned are dominantly inherited and give rise to severe central visual loss. Stargardt's disease, North Carolina macular dystrophy and Best's disease usually reduce the vision significantly before the age of 20. Sorby's macular dystrophy causes significant visual loss in the 20s to 40s. Patients with central areolar choroidal dystrophy do not usually have significant visual loss until the 50s.

47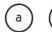

Proliferative diabetic retinopathy is the result of severe retinal ischaemia. Any condition that either reduces the number of nerve fibre layers or increases oxygen transmission between the choroidal and retinal circulation will reduce the proliferation. Renal failure is associated with hypertension and tends to exacerbate the retinal ischaemia.

46

Corneal blood staining is a complication of hyphaema. Its incidence is increased in patients with prolonged hyphaema, large hyphaema, high intraocular pressure and abnormal endothelium. Sickle cell anaemia is associated with delayed clearance of hyphaema due to sickling of the red blood cells and hence higher incidence of corneal blood staining. The use of topical steroid does not increase corneal blood staining.

48

Risk factors for corticosteroid-induced ocular hypertension include glaucoma, relatives of glaucoma patients, diabetes and myopia. The mechanism is outflow obstruction and may be caused by deposition of mucopolysaccharide in the trabecular meshwork. It is related to the potency of the steroid. Topical steroid causes ocular hypertension earlier than systemic steroids. This is due to an increased ocular concentration after topical administration compared with systemic administration. Stopping the steroid early in the course of the disease will reverse the ocular hypertension – however, irreversible ocular hypertension has been documented, especially in myopic patients.

49 The following are true about thyroid eye disease:

a   it is the commonest cause of eyelid retraction

b   it is more severe in older patients

c   it is more severe in smokers

d   its severity is related to the degree of thyrotoxicosis

e   the activity is best elucidated with STER MRI sequence.

50 The following are true about botulinum toxin:

a   the most commonly used botulinum toxin in clinical practice is type A

b   it causes irreversible post-synaptic blockage at the neuromuscular junction

c   the onset of action is about 72 hours

d   prolonged use is associated with muscle atrophy

e   in a right abducence nerve palsy, injection of botulinum into the right lateral rectus may reduce the esotropia.

51 With regard to congenital nasolacrimal duct obstruction:

a   about 6% of newborns have symptoms referrable to dacryostenosis

b   the most common site of obstruction is at the valve of Hasner

c   compression of a dacryocystocele often produces a sticky discharge through the puncta

d   early probing is recommended in patients with mucocele

e   the success rate of the initial probing is about 60%.

52 The following are true about giant cell arteritis:

a   visual loss is usually caused by ischaemia of the posterior ciliary artery

b   visual loss is usually more severe than non-arteritic optic neuropathy

c   C-reactive protein is better than ESR in monitoring the response to treatment

d   during temporal artery biopsy, the artery can be found beneath the temporalis fascia

e   the presence of skip lesion in the temporal artery is associated with a less severe form of the disease.

49

Thyroid eye disease is more common in females than males and tends to be more severe in the elderly than the young. Although hyperthyroidism occurs in about 80% of these patients, its severity does not correlate with the severity of the eye disease. STER MRI sequence is useful in detecting the activity of the disease. The presence of 'wet' sequence suggests active disease.

50

Botulinum toxin causes irreversible blockage of the pre-synaptic neurone and thus inhibits the release of acetylcholine. The onset of action is 72 hours, with a mean duration of action of 4 months. Termination of action is the result of regeneration of new dendrites. Muscle atrophy occurs in prolonged use of botulinum toxin. In right abducence nerve palsy, it can be injected into the non-paralysed muscle, i.e. the right medial rectus, to reduce contracture of the muscle and the esotropia.

51

It is estimated that congenital nasolacrimal duct obstruction occurs in 73% of newborns but only 6% are symptomatic. The most common site of obstruction is at the valve of Hasner. In a dacryocystocele, there is concurrent obstruction in the common canaliculus – therefore, compression of the sac does not show reflux. A mucocele increases the risk of orbital cellulitis and early probing is recommended. The success of first probing in congenital nasolacrimal duct obstruction approaches 90%.

52

Branches of posterior ciliary artery supply the optic nerve head. Ischaemia causes optic nerve head swelling. Compared with the non-arteritic form, the visual loss in giant cell arteritis is usually profound and more often bilateral, unless steroid treatment is carried out early. C-reactive protein is a better indicator of response to treatment because its concentration changes more quickly with the amount of inflammation. The temporal artery lies on the temporalis fascia. Skip lesion may give a negative temporal artery biopsy but does not correlate with the severity of the disease.

53 In argon laser trabeculoplasty:

a   laser is applied to the anterior half of the trabecular meshwork

b   the amount of energy used per unit area of burn is larger than in retinal photocoagulation

c   the amount of intraocular pressure reduction is related to the pre-treatment intraocular pressure

d   reduction of pressure is more marked in phakic than pseudophakic patients

e   the effect on intraocular pressure reduction becomes less with retreatment.

54 The following are true about nasolacrimal duct obstruction in the adult:

a   it is more common in females than in males

b   presence of dacryoliths occurs in 25% of patients

c   probing and syringing has a success rate of 70%

d   external DCR has a higher success rate than endonasal DCR in relieving epiphora

e   DCR involves removing most of the ethmoid bone.

55 In an eye with raised intraocular pressure caused by Sturge-Weber's syndrome, the pressure can be effectively lowered with:

a   an α blocker such as brimonidine

b   a β blocker such as timolol

c   latanoprost

d   pilocarpine

e   topical acetazolamide.

56 Laser iridotomy may be expected to reduce the intraocular pressure in:

a   phacomorphic glaucoma

b   phacolytic glaucoma

c   microspherophakia with glaucoma

d   iris bombe in severe iritis

e   malignant glaucoma following cataract surgery.

53 (a) (b) (c) (d) (e)

Argon laser trabeculoplasty increases the outflow facility of aqueous. It is applied to the anterior half of the trabecular meshwork. Application of laser to the posterior half risks the development of anterior synechiae. The effect on pressure reduction depends on the pre-treatment pressure, age of the patient and type of glaucoma. It is less effective in pseudophakic and aphakic patients. The effect of pressure reduction tends to decrease with time and retreatment tends to be less effective.

54 (a) (d)

Adult epiphora caused by nasolacrimal duct obstruction is more common in females than males. It usually occurs in post-menopausal women and there is stenosis of the nasolacrimal duct. Dacryoliths are uncommon. Unlike congenital nasolacrimal duct obstruction, syringing and probing has a low success rate. External DCR gives a higher success rate than endonasal DCR. During the operation, most of the bone removed to create a rhinostomy is from the lacrimal bone.

55 (a) (b) (c) (e)

Raised intraocular pressure in Sturge-Weber's syndrome is caused by an increase in episcleral pressure that impairs aqueous outflow. α and β blockers, as well as acetazolamide, suppress aqueous production and are therefore effective. Latanoprost is also effective as it increases the uveoscleral outflow. Pilocarpine increases the aqueous outflow through the trabecular meshwork and therefore is ineffective in the presence of raised episcleral pressure.

56 (a) (c) (d)

Laser iridotomy is used in angle-closure glaucoma caused by pupillary block by providing an alternative pathway for the aqueous. Phacomorphic glaucoma is a common contributing factor in primary angle closure. Pupillary block can be caused by the abnormal spherical lens in microspherophakia. Iris bombe impair the flow of aqueous through the pupil and hence pupillary block. Phacolytic glaucoma is caused by the release of lens proteins into the drainage angle where they are engulfed by macrophages, leading to blockage of the trabecular meshwork. Malignant glaucoma is caused by aqueous misdirection into the vitreous cavity.

57 The following are true about Tenon's cyst:

a it is caused by adhesion between the episclera and the Tenon's capsule

b it usually appears as a thick-walled lobulated mass over the trabeculectomy site

c digital pressure on the lower globe is useful in breaking the cyst

d injection of 5-fluorouracil is useful

e needling is contraindicated due to the risk of developing a persistent non-healing fistula.

58 The following steps can reduce the effect of oculocardiac reflex during operation:

a peribulbar anaesthesia

b use of suxamethonium

c use of atropine

d increasing the blood oxygen saturation

e using light sedation.

59 The following are true about exotropia:

a intermittent exotropia improves with time in the majority of cases

b intermittent exotropia usually present with diplopia

c the angle of deviation tends to be larger for distant fixation compared with near fixation

d bilateral lateral rectus recession is more effective than resect/recess surgery in basic exotropia

e overcorrection of up to 10 prism dioptres prevents recurrence of exotropia.

60 With regard to cataract extraction in eyes with uveitis:

a prophylactic systemic steroid should be given to all patients with a history of uveitis to avoid post-operative macular oedema

b posterior capsule opacification is more common compared with the general population

c acrylic implants reduce the risk of giant cell formation on the lens

d intraocular lens implant should be avoided in juvenile idiopathic arthritis

e a large capsulorrhexis is recommended.

57

Tenon's cyst results from adhesion between the episclera and Tenon's capsule, causing trapping of the aqueous. It appears as a dome-shaped mass over the operated site. Digital pressure either over it or on the lower globe may break the adhesion. If this fails, needling may be used to break the adhesion. Revision of the bleb or repeat trabeculectomy with antimetabolite agents may be required.

58

Oculocardiac reflex occurs during manipulation of the eye, especially the extraocular muscle during strabismus or retinal surgery. Both the heart rate and blood pressure drop when this happens. The use of peribulbar anaesthesia reduces the transmission of nerve impulses from the eye and therefore dampens the reflex. The use of atropine prevents bradycardia and is used to abolish the reflex. Other measures mentioned are ineffective.

59

Intermittent exotropia seldom resolves spontaneously. The majority of patients present with aesthenopia

due to the extra effort needed to hold the two eyes together or due to awareness of the strabismus. Diplopia is not usually noticed because of suppression. Intermittent exotropia tends to have a larger angle of deviation at distant compared with near fixation (basic exotropia). In basic exotropia, resect/recess surgery is the treatment of choice whereas in simulated exotropia, bilateral lateral rectus recession appears to be more effective. Initial overcorrection of up to 10 prism dioptres reduces the incidence of recurrence. The initial esotropia tends to lessen with time.

60

Prophylactic systemic steroid treatment is only recommended in patients with previous macular oedema caused by the uveitis. Post-operative uveitis and posterior capsule opacification are more common compared with the general population. To prevent deposits of materials on the lens, either an acrylic- or heparin-coated lens may be used. Lens implant in juvenile idiopathic arthritis is associated with fibrovascular proliferation over the lens and risk of phthisis bulbi. A large capsulorrhexis reduces the incidence of synechiae between the iris and the lens capsule.

61 The following are true about the development of orbital emphysema following orbital injury:

a it is most often seen in orbital floor fracture

b prophylactic antibiotic is needed to prevent orbital cellulitis

c CT scan can usually identify the location

d infraorbital nerve anaesthesia is a feature

e repair is needed in about 50% of cases.

62 The following are true about lattice degeneration:

a it is found in 8% of the general population

b the vitreous over the lesion is firmly attached to the retina

c atrophic holes within the lattice degeneration are the most common cause of retinal detachment

d about 50% of patients with retinal detachment have lattice degeneration

e sclerosed blood vessels occur within the lattice degeneration.

63 The following are true about strabismus surgery:

a during a resect/recess operation, resection should be performed before recession

b operating on the medial rectus has a more significant effect on the amount of strabismus correction compared with the lateral rectus

c a combined resect/recess operation has a greater effect than if the two procedures are carried out on separate occasions

d adjustable suture should be avoided in inferior rectus surgery

e resection of the superior rectus is associated with lid retraction.

64 The findings of the following are in favour of neurogenic rather than mechanical muscle palsy:

a duction of the affected eye results in more movement than version

b Hess chart of the affected eye is smaller

c the intraocular pressure is normal in all directions of gaze

d the absence of retraction of the globe

e abnormal head posture may be adopted to reduce diplopia.

61 (b)

Orbital emphysema usually results from medial wall fractures such that sneezing or nose-blowing forces air from the paranasal sinuses into the orbital tissue. Prophylactic antibiotic prevents orbital cellulitis. The fracture is often small and difficult to locate even with a CT scan. The majority of cases resolve spontaneously and surgery is rarely required. Infraorbital nerve anaesthesia is a feature of orbital floor fractures.

62 (a) (d) (e)

Lattice degeneration occurs in 8% of the population but only a small minority of these patients develop retinal detachment. However, it is found in 50% of patients with retinal detachment. The cause of detachment is usually due to a retinal tear surrounding the lattice degeneration, where the vitreous is firmly attached to the retina. Over the lesion, the vitreous is typically liquefied. Pigmentation and sclerosed vessels are common features within the lesion.

63 (b) (c) (d) (e)

Resection involves cutting and shortening of the muscle, whereas recession involves moving the muscle insertion to a more posterior position. Recession is reversible, whereas resection is not; therefore, recession should always be performed before resection in case of iatrogenic mishaps such as erroneous identification of the muscle. The medial rectus is stronger than the lateral rectus and, therefore, operation on this muscle has a greater effect. The inferior rectus muscle has a tendency to slip into the orbit when detached – therefore, adjustable sutures are not recommended. Superior rectus resection can cause upper lid retraction.

64 (a) (c) (d)

Duction refers to movement of one eye, whereas version refers to conjugate movement of both eyes. Because of Hering's law of equal innervation, conjugate eye movement of the affected eye is less than duction. Hess charts in both cases are reduced – however, in a neurogenic palsy, there is proportional spacing between the inner and the outer fields. Intraocular pressures are elevated in a mechanical muscle palsy when the patient looks away from the site of the mechanical lesion. Globe retraction occurs in a mechanical palsy when the patient looks away from the site of the lesion. Abnormal head posture may be adopted in both conditions.

65 The following are true about myelinated nerve fibres in the eye:

a myelination of the optic tract begins at the optic nerve head before birth

b myelination is produced by astrocytes

c it is more common in males than females

d it has no visual consequence

e spontaneous disappearance occurs in multiple sclerosis.

66 In retinal detachment caused by retinal dialysis:

a trauma is the major cause

b the most common site is the inferotemporal region

c folding of the posterior edge of the retinal dialysis is common

d the prognosis is poorer than for the patient with retinal detachment caused by retinal tear

e high scleral buckling is essential for successful closure of retinal dialysis.

67 The following are true about diabetic retinopathy:

a diabetic retinopathy is rare before the onset of puberty

b the severity of diabetic retinopathy is related to the control of diabetes mellitus

c the probability of progression from pre-proliferative to proliferative diabetic retinopathy is 50% over a 2-year period

d the major cause of visual loss in diabetic retinopathy is vitreous haemorrhage

e aspirin is useful in delaying the progression of diabetic retinopathy.

68 The following are true about retinopathy of prematurity:

a screening should be performed for all babies born with a weight of less than 1500g or less than 31 weeks of gestational age

b retinopathy of prematurity typically occurs at about 4 weeks after delivery

c rush disease refers to the presence of vitreous cells and tortuous blood vessels

d threshold disease is determined by the stage as well as the zone of the disease

e increased kappa angle is seen in patients with cicatricial stage of the disease.

65

Myelination of the optic tract begins at the lateral geniculate body and is produced by the oligodendrocytes. The incidence is about 0.3% and affects males more than females. It is associated with amblyopia and myopia. In multiple sclerosis, demyelination occurs and may cause spontaneous resolution of the condition.

66

The most common cause of retinal dialysis is trauma. The most common site is the inferotemporal region followed by the superonasal region. The posterior edge of the retinal dialysis remains attached to the vitreous base, which prevents it from curling over, unlike a giant retinal tear. Compared with retinal detachment, the prognosis for retinal dialysis is good. High buckling should be avoided during the operation as this would cause fish-mouthing and prevent closure.

67

Diabetic retinopathy occurs in 50% of patients with diabetes mellitus who have had the disease for more than 7 years. The Diabetic Control and Complications Trial shows that good diabetic control significantly reduces the incidence of diabetic retinopathy. While the visual loss from vitreous haemorrhage is often profound, the major cause of visual loss in diabetic retinopathy is macular oedema. The Early Treatment of Diabetic Retinopathy Study shows that aspirin has no effect on either non-proliferative or proliferative diabetic retinopathy.

68

Risk factors for retinopathy of prematurity (ROP) are low birth weight (<1500g) and early gestational age (<31 weeks). ROP typically occurs 6 to 8 weeks after delivery and is estimated to occur in about 5% of all premature babies. Rush disease refers to rapid progression of ROP, whereas plus disease refers to the presence of vitreous cells and tortuous blood vessels. Threshold disease is defined as stage 3 ROP with 5 or more contiguous, or 8 or more interrupted, clock hours in the presence of plus disease in zone I or II. Increased kappa angle occurs in cicatricial stages of the disease, with dragged disc causing the fovea to be displaced laterally.

69 The following features favour a diagnosis of choroidal melanoma rather than naevus:

a a height of more than 3mm on ultrasound

b high internal reflectivity on A-scan

c presence of drusen on the surface

d visual field defects

e presence of choroidal neovascular membrane.

70 The following are true about central retinal vein occlusion:

a haematological disorders are more common in patients less than 60 years of age than those over 60 years of age

b the prognosis for younger patients is better than for older patients

c the Central Retinal Vein Occlusion Study (CRVOS) shows that aspirin can prevent recurrence in the affected eye or involvement of the fellow eye

d the Central Vein Occlusion Study shows clear benefit of prophylactic laser treatment in ischaemic eyes

e grid laser photocoagulation is useful in the presence of macular oedema with a visual acuity of 6/18.

71 The following are true about the management of branch retinal vein occlusion:

a laser treatment should be carried out within 3 months from the onset of the event to be effective

b clinical diagnosis is usually sufficient to decide on the advantage of laser treatment in a patient with macular oedema

c patients with hypertension are unlikely to benefit from laser treatment

d if the vision is less than 6/60, macular laser is unlikely to be beneficial

e laser treatment should be carried out in the presence of retinal non-perfusion of 5 disc diameter or more, based on the fluorescein angiography.

69

The most important differential diagnosis of choroidal melanoma is the choroidal naevus. There are certain features that favour the diagnosis of choroidal melanoma and these include:

- a height of more than 3mm
- overlying orange pigment in the retinal pigment epithelium (lipofuscin) as compared to drusen in choroidal naevi
- presence of subretinal fluid
- high internal reflectivity on A-scan
- visual field defect.

Choroidal neovascular membrane can occur in both conditions and are of little use in differentiation.

70

In central retinal vein occlusion, haematological disorders such as protein S or C deficiency are more commonly detected in patients under the age of 60. Compared with the older age group, the visual prognosis for younger patients is better. The Central Retinal Vein Occlusion Study shows no distinct advantage of prophylactic laser treatment in ischaemic eyes provided the patients can be followed up regularly for the development of neovascularisation. The effect of aspirin was not considered in this study. Grid

photocoagulation in macular oedema with a visual acuity of 6/18 has not been found to be useful in this study.

71

Based on the findings of the Branch Retinal Vein Occlusion Study Group, laser treatment is useful in macular oedema secondary to branch retinal vein occlusion if: first, the foveal vasculature is intact and, second, the vision is between 6/12 and 6/60. Fluorescein angiography is essential in identifying patients who would benefit from laser treatment. Laser treatment should also be delayed until 3 to 6 months after the event to allow for spontaneous resolution of oedema and intraretinal haemorrhages. While retinal non-perfusion of 5 disc diameter or more increases the risk of peripheral neovascularisation, laser need not be performed provided the patients can be followed up at regular intervals.

72 In the management of cytomegalovirus (CMV) retinitis with HAART (highly active anti-retroviral therapy):

a HAART compresses steroids and gancyclovir

b HAART improves the survival rate of AIDS patients with CMV retinitis

c CMV virus is eradicated

d the risk of opportunistic infection is reduced

e severe vitritis is a complication.

73 The following are the guidelines based on the Diabetic Retinopathy Study (DRS):

a immediate laser treatment should be administered to eyes with optic disc neovascularisation, irrespective of size

b immediate laser treatment should be administered to all pregnant women with severe non-proliferative diabetic retinopathy

c pan-retinal photocoagulation should be administered in one session for maximal effect

d retinal neovascularisation should never be lasered directly

e argon laser is more effective than diode laser in retinal pan-photocoagulation.

74 The following are true for the phakomatoses and the location of their abnormal gene:

a type I neurofibromatosis – chromosome 21

b tuberous sclerosis – chromosome 9

c von Hippel-Lindau's syndrome – chromosome 3

d ataxic telangiectasia – chromosome 13

e Wyburn-Mason syndrome – X chromosome.

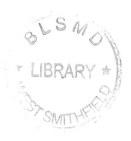

72

HAART involves the combination of anti-retroviral drugs such as nucleoside reverse transcriptase inhibitors (nucleosides), non-nucleoside reverse transcriptase inhibitors (NNRTI) and protease inhibitors (PI). It has been shown to improve the survival rate of AIDS patients with CMV retinitis. During treatment, the CD4+ T lymphocytes are increased and the risk of opportunistic infection is reduced. In addition, the time interval between relapses of CMV retinitis is increased. However, the CMV virus is not eradicated but merely suppressed. One of the commonly encountered complications of HAART is severe vitritis, thought to be caused by the restored T lymphocytes which act against the CMV virus. Vitritis can lead to cystoid macular oedema, which impairs the patient's vision.

73 **None**

The guidelines based on the DRS are as follows.

- Immediate laser treatment should be given to an eye with optic disc neovascularisation which is associated with retinal or vitreous haemorrhage, and in the absence of the latter when the extent of disc neovascularisation is at least one-quarter to one-third disc area.
- Laser treatment is also recommended for neovascularisation elsewhere which is at least one-half disc area in extent with pre-retinal or vitreous haemorrhage.
- Pan-photocoagulation should be divided into several sessions in close succession rather than in a single visit, to prevent complications such as macular oedema.
- Direct laser can be applied to flat neovascularisation elsewhere but not to disc vessels or vessels elsewhere which are elevated.

74

There are nine conditions classified under phakomatoses and their genetic loci are as follows:

- neurofibromatosis type I – autosomal dominant – chromosome 17
- type II – autosomal dominant – chromosome 22
- tuberous sclerosis – autosomal dominant – chromosome 9
- Sturge-Weber's syndrome – sporadic
- von Hippel-Lindau's syndrome – autosomal dominant – chromosome 3
- Louis-Bar syndrome–autosomal recessive – chromosome 11
- Wyburn-Mason syndrome – sporadic
- Klippel-Trenaunay-Weber syndrome – autosomal dominant – chromosome unknown
- cutis marmarata telangiectasia congenita – sporadic.

75 The following are true about systemic drugs used in the treatment of glaucoma:

a acetazolamide causes tachypnoea

b acetazolamide should be avoided in patients with hepatic failure

c mannitol should be warmed to room temperature before intravenous administration to avoid formation of crystals

d glycerol is administered by rapid intravenous infusion

e glycerol is more effective than mannitol in lowering intraocular pressure.

76 The following are true about macular holes:

a epiretinal membrane is commonly associated with macular hole

b only half of stage 1 macular holes progress

c Watzke-Allen's sign is positive in stage 1 macular hole

d posterior vitreous detachment occurs in stage 3 macular hole

e following successful macular hole surgery, cataract is a common cause of poor vision.

77 With regard to central serous retinopathy:

a it is associated with the use of inhaled steroid

b 90% show classical smoke stack appearance on fluorescein angiography

c optic disc pit is present in 25% of cases

d laser photocoagulation reduces the incidence of recurrence

e laser photocoagulation increases the risk of choroidal neovascularisation.

78 In the following conditions, there is reduction of ERG b-wave amplitude as compared to the a-wave:

a siderosis

b Best's disease

c central retinal vein occlusion

d vigabatrin toxicity

e cancer-associated retinopathy.

75

Acetazolamide causes metabolic acidosis which in turn causes tachypnoea. It should be avoided in patients with renal or hepatic failure as it can cause fatal acid-base imbalance. Mannitol is an effective osmotic diuresis and more effective than glycerol in lowering the intraocular pressure. Glycerol should not be given intravenously as it causes severe vasoconstriction of the afferent glomerular arterioles and resultant haematuria.

76

Epiretinal membrane can give rise to pseudohole and is not a feature of idiopathic macular hole. About 50% of stage 1 macular holes progress. Watzke-Allen's sign, in which a break in the slit beam is observed, occurs in full-thickness hole, usually at stage 3 and 4. Posterior vitreous detachment occurs in stage 4. Cataract is a common complication of vitrectomy and a significant cause of poor vision following macular hole surgery.

77

Central serous retinopathy gives rise to sensory retinal detachment due to an abnormality of the retinal pigment epithelium. The cause is unknown. It is more common in males than in females and is associated with a type A personality. Systemic and inhaled steroids have also been implicated. While a smoke stack is a classical picture in fluorescein angiography of this condition, it is seen in only 10% of cases. The rest give an ink blot appearance. Laser photocoagulation can speed up recovery but does not prevent recurrence. There is a small risk (2%) of inducing choroidal neovascularisation with laser.

78

Reduction of b-wave with relative normal a-wave occurs in disorders that result in a diffuse degeneration or dysfunction of cells in the inner nuclear layer (Muller or bipolar cells). Best's disease typically shows abnormal EOG and cancer-associated retinopathy causes generalised reduction of a- and b-waves.

79 The following are true about the visual evoked potential (VEP):

a   it is abnormal in patients with poor vision due to age-related macular degeneration

b   delayed P100 latency with normal visual acuity is a feature of recovered optic neuritis

c   it is useful in detecting early glaucomatous changes

d   the use of miotics can affect the result

e   ischaemic optic neuropathy causes a decrease in VEP amplitude in the presence of normal latency.

80 In albinism:

a   the number of melanocytes is usually normal

b   visual acuity is better in tyrosine-positive than tyrosine-negative oculocutaneous albinism

c   visual evoked potential is always abnormal

d   bleeding diathesis due to poor platelet aggregation is a feature of Hermansky-Pudlak syndrome

e   recurrent pyogenic infection is a feature in Chediak-Higashi syndrome.

81 In pseudoexfoliation syndrome:

a   deposition of pigment in the trabecular meshwork often precedes the appearance of dandruff-like material on the lens

b   pupil dilatation is usually poor with mydriatics

c   peripheral transillumination is a common feature

d   chronic open angle glaucoma occurs in about 50% of cases

e   raised intraocular pressure should always be treated, irrespective of visual field loss.

79

Visual evoked potential (VEP) is a cortical response to pattern or flash stimuli. The two parameters analysed are the latency and the amplitude. A delayed latency of pattern VEP is suggestive of a demyelination process. The amplitude of pattern VEP is useful, especially in children because it correlates well with visual acuity. Patients with abnormal visual acuity such as age-related macular degeneration will have abnormal VEPs. VEPs are not useful for visual field defects. In miotic pupils, the amount of retinal illumination is reduced and this can give rise to delayed latency. Therefore, it is important to standardise the testing conditions.

80

Albinism is a group of genetic disorders with hypopigmentation of the eye, skin and hair (oculocutaneous type) or the eye only (ocular type). The oculocutaneous type is inherited in an autosomal recessive fashion, and the ocular type in an X-linked fashion. Patients with pigment production, i.e. tyrosine-positive type, tend to have better vision. Visual evoked potential is abnormal and there is increased decussation of the optic nerve. Two types of syndromes have been described for oculocutaneous albinism:

- Chediak-Higashi syndrome: recurrent pyogenic infection and bleeding diathesis
- Hermansky-Pudlak syndrome: bleeding diatheses, pulmonary fibrosis, inflammatory bowel disease, renal failure and cardiomyopathy.

The bleeding diathesis in Hermansky-Pudlak syndrome is due to abnormal aggregation of platelets.

81

Pseudoexfoliation syndrome is an important cause of secondary open-angle glaucoma. Although the appearance of dandruff-like material is characteristic of this condition, the earliest sign is the deposition of pigment in the trabecular meshwork, lens and iris. Pupil dilatation is poor and cataract extraction may be difficult. Complications of cataract surgery are also increased due to weakened zonules, which can lead to zonulysis and vitreous loss. In about 50% of patients, chronic open angle glaucoma occurs. Intraocular pressures are often unstable and can lead to severe glaucoma. Therefore, any evidence of raised intraocular pressure should be treated early.

82 In progressive outer retinal necrosis (PORN):

a the disease is preceded by ophthalmic shingles in the majority of patients

b this condition is found almost exclusively in AIDS patients

c involvement of the macula occurs early in the course of the disease

d vitritis is usually severe

e intravenous acyclovir is usually effective in controlling the disease.

83 In a child who presents with leukocoria, the following features are in favour of retinoblastoma rather than toxocariasis:

a involvement of both eyes

b presence of calcification

c age of less than 2 years

d presence of hypopyon

e male sex.

84 The following are true about sympathetic ophthalmia:

a bilateral granulomatous pan-uveitis is a feature

b fluorescein angiography is useful for diagnostic purposes

c removal of the injured eye should be performed within a week to avoid this complication

d the choroid is typically thickened with occlusion of the choriocapillaris

e Dalen-Fuchs' nodules are found on the retinal side of Bruch's membrane.

82

PORN is caused by the varicella zoster virus, resulting in inflammation of the outer retina. Preceding ophthalmic shingles is not common. The disease has only been described in AIDS patients. Clinically, there is early involvement of the macula with little or no vitritis. Antiviral treatment, including acyclovir, has not been effective and severe visual loss is common.

83

Retinoblastoma can be bilateral, whereas toxocariasis has not been reported to affect both eyes. Calcification of the lesion is typically seen in retinoblastoma. Toxocariasis is acquired from ingestion of ova and tends to occur in older patients. Hypopyon from severe inflammation can occur in both diseases. There is no gender predilection for either condition.

84

Sympathetic ophthalmia occurs most commonly following a perforating injury but has been described in ophthalmic procedures such as cataract surgery and glaucoma surgery. Sympathetic ophthalmia is a clinical diagnosis. Fluorescein angiography does not show features typical of this condition. Although sympathetic ophthalmia has been reported as early as 5 days, the general consensus is to remove an injured sightless eye within 2 weeks of trauma. Thickening of the choroid is caused by cellular infiltration but the choriocapillaris are not involved. Dalen-Fuchs' nodules contain aggregates of lymphocytes and macrophages. They are found on the retinal side of Bruch's membrane. It is not pathognomonic of the condition as it is also seen in Vogt-Koyanagi-Harada's syndrome.

Quick fix

- The incidence of CMV retinitis in AIDS patients is related to the CD4 count. It is about 20% per year in AIDS patients with a CD4 count of less than 50 per cubic mm.

- HAART (Highly Active AntiRetroviral Therapy) uses a combination of antiretroviral medication which increases the CD4 count and therefore reduces the incidence of CMV retinitis.

85 With regard to acanthoamoeba keratitis:

a it is equally common in rigid gas permeable contact lens users as in soft contact lens users

b the most common types are *A hatchetti*

c swimming with contact lenses is a risk factor

d radial perineuritis is diagnostic

e the cyst wall can be visualised with ultraviolet light following staining with calcofluor white.

86 In sebaceous cell carcinoma of the eyelid:

a unilateral blepharitis is a common feature

b previous eyelid radiation is a risk factor

c the upper lid is more commonly involved than the lower lid

d compared with non-ocular sebaceous cell carcinoma, those affecting the eyelids tend to be more aggressive

e Sudan black is used to differentiate the tumour from squamous cell carcinoma.

87 In a patient with a pale optic disc, the following test may be useful in reaching a diagnosis:

a full blood count and film

b serum folate level

c colour vision test

d serum FTA Abs

e visual evoked potential.

85

Acanthoamoeba keratitis is caused by a free-living protozoan. The most common species involved are *A polyphaga* and *A castellani*. Improper disinfection of the contact lenses is a major risk factor as is swimming with contact lenses. Although both rigid gas permeable and soft contact lenses have been implicated in acanthoamoeba keratitis, the incidence is higher amongst soft contact lens users. Clinically, the condition is very painful for the amount of clinical signs seen. Initially, it can present with dendrites which can be mistaken for herpes simplex keratitis. Radial perineuritis is a characteristic and diagnostic feature. The protozoan can be visualised under ultraviolet light after staining with calcofluor white. *In vivo* visualisation can be achieved with confocal microscopy. The medium used to culture the organism is a nutrient-poor agar overlaid with *E coli*.

86

Sebaceous cell carcinoma of the upper lid is an aggressive tumour which can metastasise early. It typically presents as unilateral blepharitis or a recurrent chalazion. The upper lid is more commonly involved than the lower lid due to the larger number of meibomian glands in the upper lids. Risk factors include old age and previous radiation to the head. In a poorly differentiated tumour, it may be difficult to differentiate it from squamous cell carcinoma. However, the use of Sudan black or Oil red O can be useful as both will stain for the presence of fat in tumour cells seen in sebaceous cell carcinoma.

87

Optic atrophy is a physical sign and further tests are needed to find the underlying cause. Vitamin B_{12} deficiency is a cause of optic atrophy and a full blood count may show macrocytosis and hypersegmentation of the neutrophils. Serum folate may give the same haematological pictures but optic atrophy is not a feature of folate deficiency. Positive serum FTA Abs may suggest syphilis as a cause of the optic atrophy. Colour vision test and visual evoked potential are abnormal in optic atrophy and do not provide information about the underlying cause.

88 In essential blepharospasm:

a symptoms usually begin as excessive blinking

b symptoms usually improve during sleep

c the presence of facial grimace and retrocollic spasm constitute Meige's disease

d compression of the facial nerve by the inferior cerebellar artery is a recognised cause

e stripping of the orbicularis oculi is curative.

89 In stem cell deficiency:

a corneal cells at the limbus are absent

b the cornea is covered by cells resembling those of conjunctiva

c impression cytology reveals goblet cells

d corneal oedema is a common feature

e amniotic membrane graft is used to treat this condition.

90 The following are true about mitomycin C:

a it is isolated from a fungus

b it inhibits DNA synthesis

c it is used to prevent recurrence of pterygium following its excision

d it has an antifibrotic effect which is proportional to the concentration used

e its use in trabeculectomy is associated with a higher incidence of hypotony as compared with the use of 5-FU.

91 The following are true about adenovirus keratoconjunctivitis:

a membranous conjunctivitis causing puntal occlusion is a complication

b the keratitis is caused by viral replication within the epithelial cells

c subepithelial infiltrates typically develop about 2 weeks after the onset of conjunctivitis

d corneal neovascularisation is a late complication

e systemic acyclovir is useful in the acute stage.

88

Essential blepharospasm is characterised by bilateral orbicularis oculi and facial spasm. It usually begins as excessive blinking and may lead to functional blindness. The cause is unknown. Symptoms usually improve during sleep and are worsened under stressful circumstances. Meige's disease is essential blepharospasm with facial grimace, mouth retraction and retrocollic spasm. It suggests a dysfunction of the basal ganglia. Compression of the facial nerve by the inferior cerebellar artery is a recognised cause in hemifacial spasm. Treatment is usually with botulinum injection into the orbicularis oculi. In resistant cases, stripping of the orbicularis oculi may be effective.

89

In stem cell deficiency, the cells at the limbus are absent or defective. The result is conjunctivalisation of the corneal epithelium. Goblet cells may be present. Corneal oedema is not a feature because the endothelial function remains normal. Autograft transplant of limbal cells from the fellow eye, allograft transplant from a cadavertic eye or a living related donor, or amniotic membrane transplant has been used to treat stem cell deficiency.

90

Mitomycin C is isolated from *Streptomyces caespitosus* and acts as an alkylating agent which inhibits DNA synthesis. In ophthalmology, it is used mainly to prevent pterygium recurrence and in high-risk trabeculectomies. Mitomycin C is a more potent anti-metabolite than 5-FU and its use in glaucoma is isolated, with an increased risk of wound leak and hypotony.

91

Adenoviral keratoconjunctivitis can occasionally give rise to severe membranous conjunctivitis with punctal occlusion and symblepharon. The keratitis seen is caused by viral replication within the epithelium. With time, the keratitis progresses to subepithelial infiltration which is likely to be an immune response. Corneal neovascularisation is not a feature of this condition. Systemic acyclovir is of no use. In patients with severe keratoconjunctivitis, or those with reduced vision from the keratitis, steroids may be used with caution.

92 In vitamin A deficiency:

a the blood film often shows characteristic features

b visual loss is usually due to retinal degeneration

c lipid components of tear are usually affected early

d Bitot's spots are found only in the temporal bulbar conjunctiva

e nyctalopia usually precedes xerophthalmia.

93 Steven-Johnson's syndrome:

a is most often caused by drugs

b is characterised by formation of blisters on the skin

c may be confined to the skin

d is commonly associated with mucopurulent discharge from the eyes in the acute stage

e rarely causes long-term ocular sequelae.

94 The following mucopolysaccharidoses often give rise to corneal clouding:

a Hunter's syndrome

b Hurler's syndrome

c Morquio's syndrome

d Sanfilippo's syndrome

e Scheie's syndrome.

95 In keratoconus:

a the onset is usually in childhood

b progressive astigmatic myopia is the most common refractive change

c patients should avoid contact sport due to the risk of corneal perforation

d hydrops is an indication for early corneal graft

e corneal graft has a good success rate.

92 (e)

The blood film is normal in vitamin A deficiency. Abetalipoproteinaemia, a rare recessive disorder, is associated with vitamin A deficiency and the presence of astrocytic red blood cells in the blood film. Visual loss is usually caused by keratomalacia leading to perforation. Dry eye is often due to abnormal mucous membrane with goblet cell dysfunction. Night blindness (nyctalopia) occurs before xerophthalmia.

93 (a) (d)

Steven-Johnson's syndrome refers to acute inflammation of the skin and mucous membrane. Lesion confined to the skin is called erythema multiforme. The skin lesion typically appears as target lesions. Mucopurulent ocular discharge is common at the acute stage. Ocular complications are common and consist of dry eyes, symblepharon and eyelid malposition.

94 (b) (c) (e)

Mucopolysaccharidoses are a group of lysosomal storage diseases which are inherited in an autosomal recessive fashion with the exception of Hunter's syndrome which is X-linked. Although all of them can give rise to corneal clouding through deposition of accumulated metabolites, corneal clouding is only occasionally seen in Sanfilippo's syndrome and Hurler's syndrome.

95 (b) (e)

Keratoconus is an ectatic condition characterised by progressive thinning of the cornea. The condition usually begins at adolescence. Progressive astigmatic myopia is the most common finding. Despite the thinning, perforation is rare. Hydrop results from a break in Descemet's membrane leading to cornea swelling. With time, hydrops usually resolves, leaving behind a small scar. Compared with other inflammatory conditions, corneal graft in keratoconus has a higher success rate.

96 A man develops left trochlear nerve palsy following head injury. He is likely to experience increased vertical diplopia in the following situations:

a right gaze

b head tilt to the right

c down-gaze

d near reading

e up-gaze.

97 In a patient with Horner's syndrome, the following signs are seen:

a decreased intraocular pressure

b ptosis which improves with phenylephrine

c enophthalmos measurable with an exophthalmometer

d anisocoria which is most noticeable in bright light

e problem with accommodation.

98 The following are true about divisional oculomotor nerve palsy:

a it is more common than infranuclear third nerve palsy

b it suggests a lesion in the cavernous sinus

c superior division involvement is associated with hypotropia

d superior division involvement is associated with poor accommodation

e inferior division involvement causes mydriasis.

99 The following association with the respective eye movements are correct:

a see-saw nystagmus – lesion in the chiasm

b down beat nystagmus – Arnold-Chiari malformation

c ocular flutter – neuroblastoma

d convergence retraction nystagmus – mid-brain lesion

e pendular nystagmus – unilateral congenital cataract.

96

Following fourth cranial nerve palsy, vertical diplopia is usually worse on contralateral gaze (in this case right gaze), head tilt to the same (left) side, down-gaze (such as walking downstairs) and near reading.

97

In Horner's syndrome, the loss of sympathetic tone will decrease intraocular pressure. Ptosis improves with the sympathomimetic effect of phenylephrine. Enophthalmos is an apparent sign rather than a true one, due to updrawing of the lower lids. Anisocoria is typically more noticeable in dim light. Accommodation is normal.

Quick fix

Nystagmus of localising value include:

- down-beat nystagmus: lesion at the cervico-medullary junction

- see-saw nystagmus: lesion at the optic chiasm

- convergence-retraction nystagmus: mid-brain lesion

- internuclear ophthalmoplegia: the lesion in the medial longitudinal fasciculus is ipsilateral to the side with the adduction deficit.

98

Divisional oculomotor nerve palsy is less common than complete third nerve palsy. It suggests a lesion in the anterior cavernous sinus. Superior division involvement causes ptosis and hypotropia, whereas inferior division involvement causes exotropia, hypertropia, intorsion and mydriasis.

99

See-saw nystagmus is indicative of a lesion in the chiasmal region. Arnold-Chiari malformation can present with down beat nystagmus. Opsoclonus but not ocular flutter may be a sign of neuroblastoma. Convergence retraction nystagmus is a feature of mid-brain lesion such as pinealoma. Pendular nystagmus is a common feature in patients with poor vision due to congenital cataract, and this can be unilateral.

100 In a patient with proliferative diabetic retinopathy, vitrectomy is recommended in:

a an only eye with tractional retinal detachment nasal to the optic disc

b the presence of bilateral pre-retinal haemorrhages

c the presence of neovascularisation in the inferior arcade with pre-retinal haemorrhage, despite pan-retinal photocoagulation

d vitreous haemorrhage of more than 4 months duration in type I diabetes

e simultaneous presence of optic disc and peripheral neovascularisation with pre-retinal haemorrhages.

101 The following contraindications are correct:

a systemic acetazolamide in patients who develop Steven-Johnson's syndrome to sulphonamide

b topical timolol in patients on peripheral calcium channel blockers

c apraclonidine in patients taking monoamine oxidase inhibitors

d latanoprost in patients with skin melanoma

e pilocarpine in patients with raised intraocular pressure secondary to uveitis.

102 The following are true about ciliary body ablation:

a the procedure is painless

b it increases uveoscleral outflow of aqueous

c it decreases aqueous production by the ciliary body

d it is not effective in neovascular glaucoma

e sympathetic ophthalmia has been reported as a complication.

103 In a newborn with a cloudy cornea, the differential diagnoses should include:

a sclerocornea

b congenital hereditary endothelial dystrophy

c Peter's anomaly

d granular dystrophy

e megalocornea.

100

The indications for vitrectomy in diabetes have been outlined in the Diabetic Retinopathy Vitrectomy Study. These include tractional retinal detachment involving the fovea, non-clearing vitreous haemorrhage especially in type I diabetes; and progressive fibrovascular proliferation despite pan-retinal photocoagulation.

101

Acetazolamide is a sulphonamide derivative and can cause Steven-Johnson's syndrome in patients with reaction to either drug. Topical timolol is only contraindicated in the presence of central-acting calcium channel blockers. The concurrent use of both can lead to heart block. Apraclonidine may cause a hypertensive crisis in patients taking monoamine oxidase inhibitors. Latanoprost can increase melanin production in the iris but has not been shown to affect skin melanoma. Pilocarpine can exacerbate the breakdown of the blood aqueous barrier and is contraindicated in the uveitic patient.

102

Ciliary body ablation involves the use of a cryoprobe or a laser to destroy the ciliary body, thereby reducing aqueous production. The procedure can be painful and sympathetic ophthalmia has been reported as a complication. Overtreatment can lead to hypotony and, rarely, phthisis may develop. It is the treatment of choice in patients with poor visual prognosis, with high intraocular pressures (such as neovascular glaucoma), inadequately controlled with medication and/or surgery.

103

Granular dystrophy does not occur in the newborn but develops later. Megalocornea occurs when the cornea in the neonate is 12mm or more in diameter – it is associated with corneal cloudiness. A useful mnemonic for neonatal corneal opacity is STUMPED: **S**clerocornea, **T**ear in Descemet's membrane (congenital glaucoma or trauma), **U**lcer (infections), **M**etabolic (mucopolysaccharidoses), **P**osterior corneal defects (posterior keratoconus or Peters' anomaly), **E**ndothelial dystrophies (congenital hereditary stromal, posterior polymorphous dystrophy or congenital hereditary endothelial dystrophy), **D**ermoid.

104 The following are true about intraocular pressure measurement with the applanation tonometer:

a   following LASIK surgery, the IOP reading may be inaccurately high

b   excessive fluorescein may give an inaccurately high reading

c   pressure may be falsely elevated in the presence of increased corneal thickness

d   myopia may give an inaccurately low pressure measurement due to decreased rigidity of the eyeball

e   breath holding may give a low pressure reading.

105 The following are true about perimetry:

a   the peripheral visual field is better tested with Goldmann perimetry rather than Humphrey perimetry

b   both cataract and miosis can cause decreased sensitivity

c   short-term fluctuation is used in Humphrey perimetry to test the reliability of the subject

d   a contracted visual field is encountered if the correcting lens is placed too far from the eye

e   a normal visual field excludes the presence of glaucoma.

106 The following are true about normal tension glaucoma:

a   brain scan reveals a cause in about 10% of patients

b   optic nerve meningioma is a cause of normal tension glaucoma

c   a dense paracentral scotoma encroaching upon fixation is a common finding

d   the use of betaxolol has been shown to delay progression

e   a reduction of more than 30% of intraocular pressure has been shown to delay the progression of visual field defect.

107 The following are true about Down's syndrome:

a   genetic analysis invariably shows trisomy 21

b   discrete lens opacities in the anterior and posterior cortex are common

c   Brushfield's spots are more commonly seen in blue than brown irides

d   hypermetropia is a common finding

e   keratoconus with a tendency to developing hydrops is a recognised association.

104

With applanation tonometry, increased corneal thickness gives an inaccurately high reading, whereas decreased thickness gives an inaccurately low reading such as following LASIK. Myopia does not affect the reading with an applanation tonometer as with an indentation tonometer. Excessive fluorescein causes wide mires which may give falsely high readings. Breath holding increases the episcleral venous pressure and may result in a higher pressure measurement.

105

The Goldmann perimetry covers a wider visual field than Humphrey field tests which only test the central 30 degrees of visual field. Decreased sensitivity occurs in cataract, miosis, fatigue and old age. Short-term fluctuation analyses the response of the patient to the same stimulus at the same location to assess reliability. The visual field is contracted if the correcting lens is placed too far in front of the patient's eye. Glaucoma may still be present despite a normal visual field because visual field defects occur only in the presence of significant nerve fibre loss.

106

By definition, normal tension glaucoma is diagnosed after excluding other causes. Optic nerve meningioma causes compressive optic neuropathy. Brain scan seldom reveals a cause in most cases of normal tension glaucoma. A dense paracentral scotoma encroaching upon fixation is a common finding. Although betaxolol has been shown to be neuroprotective in animal models, there has been no convincing evidence which proves its use in delaying progression in normal tension glaucoma. The Collaborative Normal Tension Glaucoma Study found that reducing IOP by greater than 30% delayed the rate of visual field progression.

107

Down's syndrome is often caused by trisomy 21 but in a small minority it can result from chromosomal translocation without an increase in chromosome numbers. Cataract with snowflake opacities in the cortex, keratoconus with a tendency to developing hydrops, high myopia and esotropia are associated with Down's syndrome. Brushfield's spots are made up of aggregates of iris stromal fibres. They are more commonly seen in blue irides than brown irides.

108 In aniridia:

a there is complete absence of iris structure

b poor vision usually results from excessive photophobia

c limbal stem cell deficiency with corneal neovascularisation is a feature

d Wilm's tumour is most commonly seen in sporadic cases

e lens subluxation is a feature.

109 In a patient with peripheral bone-spicule pigmentation, the following tests are useful:

a serum ACE concentration

b serum phytanic acid

c plasma ornithine level

d plasma lipoprotein B

e urine glycosaminoglycans.

110 The following are true about the findings of the Diabetes Control and Complications Trial (DCCT):

a good diabetic control in type II diabetes reduces the risk of diabetic retinopathy

b hypoglycaemia is common in patients on intensive diabetic treatment

c good diabetic control reduces diabetic nephropathy by 50%

d there is no significant difference in the incidence of diabetic neuropathy between patients on standard and intensive diabetic treatment

e the risk of cardiovascular diseases is reduced in patients on intensive diabetic treatment.

111 In an infant with poor vision, initial constriction of pupils to darkness occurs in:

a Tay-Sachs' disease

b achromatopsia

c Leber's congenital amaurosis

d X-linked congenital stationary night blindness

e optic atrophy.

108

In aniridia, there is a remnant of iris tissue. The main cause of poor vision is foveal hypoplasia. Other associated features include glaucoma and limbal stem cell failure with an increased risk of corneal neovascularisation. Wilm's tumour is most often seen in familial cases, especially in those with abnormalities of chromosome 11. The zonules are weak and lens subluxation is common.

109

Serum ACE is useful for sarcoidosis but bone-spicule pigmentation is not seen in sarcoidosis. Serum phytanic acid is raised in Refsum's disease. Elevated ornithine level occurs in gyrate atrophy which is choroidoretinal atrophy. Plasma lipoprotein B is absent in abetalipoproteinaemia, a cause of bone-spicule pigmentation. Urine glycosaminoglycans are elevated in mucopolysaccharidoses such as Hunter's or Hurler's syndrome, in which bone-spicule pigmentation is a feature.

110

The DCCT is a clinical study conducted from 1983 to 1993 by the National Institute of Diabetes and Digestive and Kidney Diseases. The study showed that keeping blood glucose levels as close to normal as possible delays the onset and progression of eye, kidney and nerve disease caused by diabetes. In fact, it demonstrated that any sustained lowering of blood glucose helps, even if the person has a history of poor control. The study involved only type I diabetics and did not look at cardiovascular risks.

111

In Tay-Sachs' disease and optic atrophy, the pupils dilate in response to darkness. In Leber's congenital amaurosis, pupillary response is sluggish but the pupil still dilates in response to darkness.
In achromatopsia and X-linked congenital stationary night blindness, there is an initial constriction of pupils to darkness.

112 In juvenile chronic arthritis, the risk of developing uveitis is highest if:

a   the age of onset is less than 6 years of age

b   the gender is female

c   serum anti-nuclear antibodies are positive

d   more than four joints are affected

e   HLA-B27 is positive.

113 In congenital nystagmus:

a   vision decreases on convergence

b   the intensity of nystagmus increases with fixation

c   nystagmus is enhanced when one eye is covered

d   absence of nystagmus in the dark is a feature

e   the vertical optokinetic response is normal.

114 The following are true about neurofibromatosis:

a   Lisch's nodules are composed of melanocytic hamartoma

b   Lisch's nodules are diagnostic of type I neurofibromatosis

c   bilateral acoustic neurofibromas are more common in type I than type II neurofibromatosis

d   pulsatile exophthalmos is a feature of type I neurofibromatosis

e   posterior subcapsular cataract is a feature of type II neurofibromatosis.

115 In sarcoidosis:

a   serum ACE concentration is a good reflection of the activity of the disease

b   pulmonary function test shows an obstructive pattern

c   Mantoux test is typically positive in those with previous BCG vaccination

d   band keratopathy usually results from recurrent anterior uveitis

e   neurosarcoidosis is more common in the presence of retinal periphlebitis.

112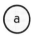

Uveitis develops in about 20% of patients with juvenile chronic arthritis. The risk is highest in the female gender, patients less than 6 years of age, pauci-ariticular joint involvement (fewer than four joints affected) and the presence of positive anti-nuclear antibodies.

113

In congenital nystagmus, vision improves on convergence and therefore vision is always better for near than distance. The intensity of the nystagmus increases with fixation. Latent nystagmus is common and closing one eye may enhance the nystagmus. Congenital nystagmus is absent in sleep but present in the dark when both eyes are open. There is an inverse horizontal optokinetic response but the vertical optokinetic response is normal.

114

Both type I and type II neurofibromatosis are autosomal dominant in inheritance. Lisch's nodules occur in type I neurofibromatosis and are composed of melanocytic hamartoma. Pulsatile exophthalmos is seen in type I neurofibromatosis caused by the absence of the lesser wing of the sphenoid bone. Type II neurofibromatosis is characterised by acoustic neuroma which may be bilateral. Posterior subcapsular cataract is also a feature.

115

Serum ACE concentration is often elevated in active sarcoidosis and its concentration reflects the activity of the disease. Pulmonary fibrosis is a complication giving a restrictive pattern on pulmonary function test. Skin anergy is common and the Mantoux test may be negative in those with previous BCG vaccination. Band keratopathy usually results from hypercalcaemia. The presence of retinal periphlebitis increases the risk of neurosarcoidosis.

116 In myasthenia gravis:

a the Tensilon test causes ventricular tachycardia

b tendon reflexes are reduced

c anti-acetylcholine receptor antibodies are more commonly detected in generalised disease than ocular myasthenia

d application of ice to a ptotic lid will reduce the ptosis

e excision of the thymus should be carried out in patients with ptosis not responding to anticholinesterase or steroid.

117 In unilateral facial nerve palsy:

a corneal sensation is reduced

b ipsilateral absence of taste in the anterior two-thirds of the tongue suggests a lesion in the facial canal

c the eye is not involved if the lesion involves the upper motor neurone

d there is retraction of the ipsilateral upper eyelid

e there is a higher chance of recovery for Ramsay Hunt's syndrome compared with Bell's palsy.

118 Intraocular foreign bodies made up of the following are relatively inert:

a aluminium

b gold

c copper

d silver

e platinum.

119 The types of giant cells seen in the following conditions are correct:

a chalazion – foreign body giant cells

b sarcoidosis – Langhans' giant cells

c juvenile xanthogranuloma – Touton giant cells

d tuberculosis – foreign body giant cells

e xanthoma disseminatum – Touton giant cells.

116

The Tensilon test can give rise to bradycardia, thus intravenous atropine should be readily available during the test. Tendon reflexes are normal in myasthenia gravis. Although antibody to acetylcholine receptors may be detected in about 80 to 90% of generalised myasthenia gravis, only 50% of pure ocular myasthenia is positive for this antibody. Ice packs can transiently improve muscle activity and therefore alleviate ptosis. Excision of the thymus is not recommended in pure ocular myasthenia gravis unless a thymoma is present.

117

The trigeminal nerve is responsible for corneal sensation. Absence of taste suggests that the lesion is in the geniculate body which is located in the middle ear. In upper motor neurone lesion of the facial nerve, the upper face including the eye is not affected, due to bilateral innervation of the upper face. Retraction of the levator results from the unopposed action of the paralysed orbicularis oculi. Facial nerve recovery is poor for Ramsay Hunt's syndrome but excellent in Bell's palsy.

118

Gold, silver and platinum are relatively inert and cause little reaction. Aluminium causes a variable amount of reaction. Copper is toxic and in high concentration (85% or above) may cause a sterile suppurative endophthalmitis.

119

There are three types of giant cells:

- Langhans' giant cells are seen in tuberculosis and sarcoidosis
- foreign body giant cells are seen in chalazion
- Touton giant cells are seen in juvenile xanthogranuloma, xanthoma disseminatum and Erdheim-Chester's disease.

Quick fix

- In foreign body giant cells, nuclei are arranged in a haphazard fashion.

- In Langhan's giant cells, nuclei are arranged in a horseshoe fashion.

- In Touton giant cells, clear cytoplasm is a feature due to the presence of cholesterol.

120 Orbital rhabdomyosarcoma:

a has a peak incidence at 10 years of age

b commonly arises from the medial rectus

c is most commonly of the alveolar type

d contains cells with a high nuclear-cytoplasmic ratio

e usually presents with fever, making it indistinguishable from orbital cellulitis.

121 Cyclosporin:

a is insoluble in water

b is excreted unchanged by the kidneys

c depresses CD4+ but not CD8+ lymphocyte function

d should be avoided in patients with anaemia as it can affect haematopoiesis

e effect can be increased with the concurrent use of ketoconazole.

122 In internuclear ophthalmoplegia:

a multiple sclerosis is the most common cause in young people

b diplopia is not a problem

c patients usually complain of problems with close work

d the lesion is ipsilateral to the eye with abducting nystagmus

e involvement of the sixth nerve nucleus is common.

123 In peribulbar anaesthesia:

a the patient should be instructed to look up to avoid perforation of the globe

b the superonasal quadrant should be avoided because of the risk of retrobulbar haemorrhage

c the risk of complications is lower with a longer needle

d the risk of complications is lower with a fine needle

e globe perforation causes increased vitreous pressure.

120

The most common age of presentation for orbital rhabdomyosarcoma is 7–8 years of age. It commonly arises from mesenchymal tissue external to the extraocular muscles. Occasionally the tumour may arise from the conjunctiva. There are three types of orbital rhabdomyosarcoma: embryonal, alveolar and differentiated. Histologically, the tumour cells have a high nuclear-cytoplasmic ratio with little cytoplasm. As a result, special tests such as immunostaining or electron-microscopy are needed for diagnosis. The tumour may be misdiagnosed as orbital cellulitis, but unlike cellulitis, fever is absent.

121

Cyclosporin is now commonly used as second-line treatment in patients with severe uveitis. It is also used in patients with high-risk corneal graft. It is lipophilic and insoluble in water. It depresses the function of CD4+ lymphocytes but has no effect on CD8+ lymphocytes. Compared with other immunosuppressants, it does not affect bone marrow function. It is metabolised by the liver and its effect is enhanced in the presence of P450 inhibitors such as ketoconazole.

122

Internuclear ophthalmoplegia may be unilateral or bilateral. In young patients, the most common cause is multiple sclerosis, whereas in the elderly, cerebrovascular accidents are more common. Rarely, tumour may be the cause. There is failure of adduction in one eye with abducting nystagmus in the fellow eye but convergence is normal. Diplopia occurs when the patient looks sideways due to the adduction deficit. Close work does not usually pose a problem because convergence is normal. The location of the lesion is in the medial longitudinal fasciculus ipsilateral to the eye with the adduction deficit. Involvement of the sixth nerve nucleus constitutes the one-and-a-half syndrome.

123

For safe peribulbar anaesthesia, the patient should keep the eye in the primary position. The superonasal and inferonasal quadrants contain a rich vascular supply and injection into these sites may be associated with an increased risk of retrobulbar haemorrhage. The use of shorter and finer needles helps to minimise complications through injuries of the nerves and vessels. Globe perforation results in hypotony.

124 The following are true about posterior capsular thickening:

a   it occurs in 50% of post-cataract patients over a 5-year period

b   it is more common in younger patients

c   it is more common in patients with diabetic retinopathy

d   it is caused by multiplication of the epithelial cells

e   it can be prevented by vigorous polishing of the posterior capsule.

125 The following are recognised features of ophthalmic herpes zoster:

a   haemorrhagic glaucoma

b   myositis

c   par planitis

d   ocular hypertension in the presence of anterior uveitis

e   diffuse iris atrophy.

126 In a patient presenting with dendritic ulcers, the following suggest that the lesion may not be caused by herpes simplex:

a   presence of uveitis

b   absence of sensation

c   absence of terminal bulbs

d   presence of ring infiltrates

e   staining with rose bengal.

127 The pairings of the following head posture and the respective ocular motility disorders are correct:

a   right sixth nerve palsy – face turn to the right

b   right fourth nerve palsy – head tilt to the right

c   bilateral fourth nerve palsy – chin depression

d   bilateral superior rectus palsy – chin elevation

e   chronic progressive external ophthalmoplegia – chin elevation.

124

Posterior capsule thickening can significantly reduce visual acuity. It is usually caused by migration of the epithelial cells to the posterior pole and multiplication of the epithelial cells. It is more common in younger patients, in diabetic retinopathy and uveitis. Polishing of the posterior capsule does not prevent opacity from developing, as epithelial cells can still migrate from the anterior capsule.

125

Follicular conjunctivitis and episcleritis are common in patients with ophthalmic herpes zoster. Intraocular complications are most common in those with nasociliary involvement. These can include keratitis, uveitis, vasculitis and myositis. Uveitis may be associated with hypopyon and haemorrhage; trabeculitis is common and may give rise to troublesome glaucoma. Iris atrophy can occur as a result of vasculitis and this is typically sectorial rather than diffuse.

126

Most dendritic ulcers are caused by herpes simplex. Two conditions that can mimic herpetic dendrites are herpes zoster keratitis and early stages of acanthoamoeba. In both cases the characteristic terminal bulbs of herpetic dendrites are absent. In acanthoamoeba, the pain is usually disproportionate to the clinical appearance of the lesion. Other features of acanthoamoeba keratitis include ring infiltrates and perineural infiltrates. Decreased corneal sensation, variable amount of uveitis and staining of the lesion with rose bengal are common features of herpetic dendritis.

127

Abnormal head posture is adopted by patients to maintain binocular single vision. In a sixth nerve palsy, the face is turned in the direction of the affected eye. In a fourth nerve palsy, the head tilt is opposite to the side of the lesion. Chin depression is seen in bilateral fourth nerve palsy and less commonly in bilateral inferior rectus palsy. Chin elevation occurs with ptosis as in chronic progressive external ophthalmoplegia and superior rectus palsy.

128 The following are true about ptosis surgery:

a   in involutional ptosis, levator resection is seldom required

b   in a patient with right amblyopia and an ipsilateral congenital ptosis covering the pupil, unilateral brow suspension is the treatment of choice

c   in ptosis due to chronic progressive external ophthalmoplegia, levator resection is the treatment of choice

d   ptosis surgery should never be performed on patients with myasthenia gravis

e   in Marcus-Gunn jaw-winking ptosis, unilateral lid surgery is usually unsatisfactory.

129 In sickle cell disease:

a   HbSC and HbSThal are more likely to cause proliferative retinopathy than HbSS

b   degenerative retinoschisis is commonly seen in the superotemporal quadrant

c   an increased foveal avascular zone with microaneurysms is a cause of poor vision

d   proliferative vitreoretinopathy most commonly affects the peripheral retina

e   blood transfusion reduces the severity of the retinopathy.

130 Benign intracranial hypertension:

a   is a complication of treatment for acne

b   does not give rise to focal neurological deficits

c   typically shows dilated ventricles on the CT scan

d   requires optic nerve fenestration to be performed prophylactically to prevent optic nerve damage

e   is unlikely to be the diagnosis if there are hard exudates at the macula.

128

The choice of ptosis surgery depends on the function of the levator. In involutional ptosis, the levator function is good and therefore only advancement is required. In the presence of amblyopia and severe ptosis, unilateral brow suspension is usually not satisfactory because the patient may not use the frontalis muscle to lift the eye due to amblyopia. The choice of surgery is disinsertion of the contralateral eye followed by bilateral brow suspension. In chronic progressive external ophthalmoplegia, levator resection may lead to corneal exposure when the function of the orbicularis oculi weakens with time. Brow suspension is the recommended technique. Although myasthenia gravis can cause ptosis, persistent ptosis may develop which is unresponsive to systemic cholinesterase treatment. Surgery may be performed provided the ptosis has been recorded as being stable for about 1 year. In Marcus-Gunn jaw-winking syndrome, unilateral ptosis surgery does not abolish the winking. Bilateral levator disinsertions followed by brow suspension is recommended.

129

In sickle cell disease, HbSC and HbSThal are most commonly

associated with severe proliferative retinopathy despite a benign systemic course. Retinoschisis occurs as a result of resorption of intraretinal haemorrhage. Occlusion of capillaries causes an increased foveal avascular zone and microaneurysms may be seen, especially with fluorescein angiography. Proliferative retinopathy is an important cause of visual loss through vitreous haemorrhage and retinal detachment. The new vessels usually occur in the peripheral retina. Blood transfusion does not affect the retinopathy.

130

Benign intracranial hypertension typically affects females who are obese. Patients on tetracycline or steroid may also develop this condition. The diagnosis is made after excluding other causes of raised intracranial hypertension. There should be no focal neurological deficit, although false localising signs such as sixth nerve palsy may be present. Optic nerve fenestration is indicated in progressive visual field loss despite repeated removal of the cerebrospinal fluid. Macular exudate may develop, causing visual disturbance.

131 The following are true about the management of cytomegaloviral (CMV) retinitis:

a zidovudine (AZT) is not effective against CMV retinitis

b the main complication of gancyclovir is bone marrow toxicity

c the main complication of foscarnet is nephrotoxicity

d viral resistance to gancyclovir will also prevent the effective use of foscarnet

e intravitreal administration of gancyclovir or foscarnet will avoid systemic complications.

132 Glycosylated haemoglobin assay:

a reflects red blood cell exposure to glucose in the last six weeks

b is used in the diagnosis of diabetes mellitus

c correlates with the risk of development of microvascular disease

d is artificially high in a patient with sickle cell anaemia

e if low in diabetes mellitus can be associated with hypoglycaemia.

133 In Marfan's syndrome:

a blood test is useful for diagnosis

b there is a point mutation in the long arm of chromosome 15

c the majority of cases are the result of a new mutation

d lens subluxation is in the superonasal direction

e myopia is common.

134 In a patient with sudden onset of visual loss, the following favour the diagnosis of ophthalmic artery over central retinal artery occlusion:

a absent a- and b-wave on the ERG

b absent cherry red spot

c relative afferent pupillary defect

d visual acuity of light perception

e delayed choroidal circulation during fluorescein angiography.

131

AZT is not effective against CMV retinitis. The three drugs most commonly used are gancyclovir, foscarnet and cidofovir. Gancyclovir causes bone marrow toxicity, whereas foscarnet and cidofovir cause nephrotoxicity. Viral resistance to one drug does not prevent the use of another to be effective. In patients with systemic complications, intravitreal drugs can be given.

132

Glycosylated haemoglobin reflects red blood cell exposure to glucose in the last six weeks. It is used to assess diabetic control. It is not used to diagnose diabetes mellitus. It correlates well with the risk of microvascular disease. In sickle cell anaemia, the concentration may be artificially low. A low level in a diabetic may indicate that the patient is predisposed to recurrent hypoglycaemia.

133

Marfan's syndrome is a clinical diagnosis. The point mutation is in the fibrillin gene on the long arm of chromosome 15. The majority of cases are inherited and only 15% are caused by new mutations. Ocular manifestations include myopia and ectopia lentis with superonasal subluxation of the lens.

134

In ophthalmic artery occlusion, the visual loss is usually profound and vision is typically light perception or worse, as opposed to counting finger vision in central retinal artery occlusion. As the choroidal circulation is affected, cherry red spot is absent. The ERG in central retinal artery occlusion shows a decreased b-wave amplitude and a relatively normal a-wave; in ophthalmic artery occlusion, both a- and b-wave are absent. Relative afferent pupillary defect is present in both conditions but is usually more marked in ophthalmic artery occlusion.

135 In a patient with proptosis, the following features favour a lesion in the orbital apex rather than the cavernous sinus:

a decreased vision with relative afferent pupillary defect

b abduction deficit

c dilated pupil

d absent forehead sensation

e loss of sensation in the lower eyelid.

136 The following are true about photodynamic therapy:

a it is effective in both classic and occult choroidal neovascularisation

b indocyanine green angiography is essential before commencement of treatment

c retinal pigment epithelial detachments are not suitable for treatment

d therapy works by causing proliferation of the retinal pigment epithelium

e argon laser is used.

137 In carotid artery stenosis:

a the atheroma is most commonly found at the bifurcation of the common carotid artery

b the bruit, if present, is best heard opposite the thyroid gland

c the risk of stroke is higher with cerebral TIAs (transient ischaemic attacks) than with ocular TIAs

d endarterectomy is superior to medical treatment in the prevention of stroke in a patient with moderate stenosis

e the addition of dipyridamole to aspirin has no additive effect in reducing the risk of stroke.

135

The optic nerve does not pass through the cavernous sinus and therefore the presence of a relative afferent pupillary defect suggests a lesion in the orbital apex.

An abduction deficit is caused by a sixth nerve palsy, a dilated pupil by a third nerve lesion and absent forehead sensation by an ophthalmic nerve lesion. All the aforementioned structures pass through both the cavernous sinus and the orbital apex. Loss of sensation in the lower eyelid is caused by maxillary nerve involvement and suggests a lesion in the cavernous sinus because this nerve does not enter the orbital apex.

136

In photodynamic therapy, a photosensitive dye such as verteporfin is injected which is then taken up by the endothelium of the choroidal neovascularisation. Infra-red laser is used to irradiate these vessels causing damage to the endothelium but sparing the retinal pigment epithelium and the photoreceptors. Only classic choroidal neovascularisation is suitable for treatment; patients with haemorrhage and retinal pigment epithelial detachment are not suitable for treatment.

137

Carotid artery stenosis can give rise to recurrent TIAs and stroke. The stenosis caused by an atheroma is found usually at the bifurcation of the common carotid artery. The bruit is best heard over the angle of the jaw. The annual risk of stroke is 8% for cerebral TIAs and 2% for ocular TIAs. However, the cause of death is usually myocardial infarction rather than stroke. Endarterectomy is superior to medical treatment in symptomatic cases with significant stenosis of over 70%.
Endarterectomy has not been shown to be advantageous over medical treatment in moderate stenosis of between 50 and 60%. Aspirin is the medication of choice. Dipyridamole can be given as an alternative but has no additive effect.

Quick fix

- The benefit of photodynamic therapy (PDT) is shown in the TAP study (*Photodynamic therapy of subfoveal choroidal neovascularisation in age-related macular degeneration with verteporfin*).

- PDT reduces visual loss from subfoveal subretinal neovascularisation caused by age-related macular degeneration.

138 With regard to the following visual field defects:

a   a right temporal lesion causes a left superior homonymous quadrantanopia

b   a left superior occipital lesion causes a right inferior homonymous quadrantanopia

c   a junctional scotoma comprises a central scotoma in one eye and superotemporal field loss in the other

d   a junctional scotoma is a feature of Kennedy-Foster's syndrome

e   bitemporal hemianopia from a pituitary lesion usually begins superiorly.

139 The following are true when assessing patients for cataract surgery:

a   patients with Fuch's heterochromic cyclitis should only undergo surgery if there is an absence of cells in the anterior chamber for at least one week

b   patients with significant diabetic macular oedema should undergo laser photocoagulation before cataract surgery

c   patients with lattice degeneration and atrophic holes should undergo cryotherapy before cataract surgery

d   an active herpetic lesion of the cornea is a contraindication to surgery

e   a dacryocystorhinostomy should be performed in the presence of a nasolacrimal duct obstruction prior to cataract surgery.

140 The following are true of endophthalmitis which developed 2 years post-trabeculectomy:

a   it does not occur in the absence of a leaking bleb

b   it is associated with the use of 5-fluorouracil

c   it is most commonly caused by *Staphylococcus*

d   it has a benign course compared with other forms of post-operative endophthalmitis

e   it can be effectively treated with intensive topical antibiotics.

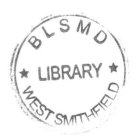

138

A temporal lobe lesion causes a superior homonymous quadrantanopia, whereas a parietal lobe lesion causes an inferior homonymous quadrantanopia. Lesion in the occipital lobe causes homonymous hemianopia, and a lesion in the lower occipital lobe causes superior homonymous quadrantanopia. A junctional scotoma is caused by a lesion at the junction between the optic nerve and the optic chiasm, resulting in the compression of the knee of Wilbrand. The visual field defect is made up of an ipsilateral central scotoma and a contralateral superotemporal field defect. Chiasmal lesions from a pituitary lesion typically present with early superior field loss.

139

In Fuch's heterochromic cyclitis, cells in the anterior chamber do not respond to steroid and their presence should not result in postponement of cataract surgery. However, Fuch's heterochromic cyclitis is associated with certain operative complications due to poor pupillary dilatation and a tendency for the iris to bleed (Amsler's sign). Patients with proliferative diabetic retinopathy and significant macular oedema should undergo laser treatment prior to cataract surgery. In maculopathy, it is recommended that laser is performed 12 weeks before cataract surgery. Retinal detachment following cataract surgery is usually the result of a fresh retinal tear. Prophylactic treatment of lattice degeneration and atrophic holes is not necessary. Active ocular infections, including herpetic keratitis, is a contraindication to cataract surgery. Nasolacrimal duct obstruction in the absence of a mucocele is not a contraindication to cataract surgery.

140

Infection can enter the eye through a microscopic break in the absence of an obvious leaking bleb. A thin cystic bleb such as those created with the use of mitomycin C or 5-fluorouracil increases the risk of infection. The most commonly isolated pathogens are *Streptococcus* and *Haemophilus*. The endophthalmitis can cause severe visual loss unless treated early. The management should include a vitreous tap for culture and sensitivity and intravitreal antibiotics.

141 The following are true about limbal dermoids:

a   they are hamartomas

b   they are most commonly found in the inferotemporal region

c   limbal dermoids are more commonly associated with systemic diseases than orbital dermoids

d   limbal dermoids give a plus cylinder with an axis along the meridian of the lesion

e   early removal of limbal dermoids will prevent refractive amblyopia.

142 Acoustic neuromas:

a   arise from the vestibular nerve of the eighth cranial nerve

b   are benign tumours of Schwann cell origin

c   cause a reduced blink reflex

d   commonly present with facial nerve palsy

e   are a feature of neurofibromatosis type II.

143 Orbital lymphomas:

a   most often arise from the lacrimal fossa

b   should not be biopsied due to the risk of tumour dissemination

c   are of high-grade non-Hodgkins' lymphoma in the majority of cases

d   usually have systemic involvement at presentation

e   are best treated with radiotherapy.

144 The following organisms can penetrate an intact cornea:

a   *Staphylococcus aureus*

b   *Pseudomonas aeruginosa*

c   *Neisseria gonorrhoea*

d   *Corynebacterium diphtheriae*

e   *Escherichia coli.*

141

Limbal dermoids are choristomas, i.e. proliferation of normal tissue in abnormal locations. They are most commonly located in the inferotemporal region. Systemic diseases such as Goldenhar's syndrome are an association. They often induce oblique astigmatism with a plus cylinder axis along the meridian of the lesion. Despite early removal, the astigmatism usually remains. Some refractive amblyopia is present even with spectacle correction.

142

Acoustic neuromas, despite the name, arise from the vestibular nerve of the eighth cranial nerve. The most common location is the internal auditory canal. The tumour is made up of benign Schwann cells. Acoustic neuromas can cause compression of the fifth or seventh cranial nerve, resulting in a reduced or abnormal blink reflex. Facial nerve palsy is a rare presentation. Most patients present with neurosensory deafness, disequilibrium or tinnitus.

143

The lacrimal fossa is the most common location (about 50%) for orbital lymphoma. Biopsy is essential for diagnosis. The majority of orbital lymphomas are of low grade and do not show systemic dissemination at presentation. However, long-term follow-up is essential because of the risk of systemic involvement. Radiotherapy is the treatment of choice.

144

Bacteria that can penetrate an intact cornea include *Neisseria gonorrhoea*, *Nesseria meningitidis* and *Corynebacterium diphtheriae*.

145 The following are true about cataract seen in congenital rubella:

a nuclear sclerosis is a feature

b microspherophakia is a feature of rubella cataract

c the rubella virus can be isolated from the lens content

d retention of lens fibre nuclei is a feature

e it is a common cause of glaucoma in congenital rubella.

146 Endothelial proliferation is a feature of:

a congenital hereditary endothelial dystrophy

b iridocorneal endothelial syndrome

c chronic uveitis

d traumatic angle recession

e posterior polymorphous dystrophy.

147 The following are indications for surgery in a blow out fracture:

a cosmetically unacceptable enophthalmos

b fracture involving more than 50% of the floor

c diplopia on up-gaze

d anaesthesia of the lower lid

e hyphaema.

148 In a patient with an alkaline burn:

a the eye should be irrigated immediately until the pH is about 7.5

b calcium hydroxide (lime) causes more damage than sodium hydroxide

c limbal ischaemia is used to decide on the severity of the damage

d conjunctival erythema is associated with poor visual prognosis

e topical steroids are contraindicated due to the risk of perforation.

145

Bilateral or unilateral cataracts are common in congenital glaucoma. The cataract typically involves the nucleus but white cataracts are also commonly seen. The lens tends to be small and spherical. The rubella virus has been isolated from lens material years after birth. Cataract extraction may release the virus, resulting in endophthalmitis. Retention of lens fibre nuclei is common. Glaucoma often co-exists with cataract but is not caused by the cataract.

146

Congenital hereditary endothelial dystrophy is characterised by absent or atrophic endothelium, resulting in corneal oedema. Chronic uveitis does not cause endothelial proliferation. Endothelial proliferation occurs in iridocorneal endothelial syndrome, traumatic angle recession and posterior polymorphous dystrophy. This proliferation can involve the trabecular meshwork, giving rise to glaucoma.

147

Repair of the blow out fracture is indicated in:

- cosmetically unacceptable enophthalmos
- a large fracture
- entrapment of the inferior rectus
- presence of diplopia in the primary position.

148

Immediate irrigation is essential until the pH is about 7.5. Lime causes less damage to the eye than sodium hydroxide or ammonium hydroxide. The presence of limbal ischaemia is an indication of the severity of the injury and can predict the extent of stem cell loss. Conjunctival erythema is common and does not affect the visual prognosis. Steroids should be used cautiously due to the risk of sterile ulceration and, occasionally, perforation.

149 In a child with accommodative esotropia:

a the condition can usually be detected at birth

b cycloplegic refraction is required to avoid under-estimation of the hypermetropia

c the amount of hypermetropia is usually greater than 1.5D

d the presence of inferior oblique overaction does not support the diagnosis

e strabismus surgery may be an option instead of glasses to correct the esotropia.

150 The following are true statements about ocular complications of ionising radiation:

a α radiation has a deeper tissue penetration than β radiation

b true exfoliation of the lens is a feature

c corneal perforation can result from dry eye and limbal stem cell failure

d the retina is more sensitive to radiation than the lens

e radiation retinopathy is caused chiefly by damage to photoreceptors.

151 The following are true about Nd:YAG capsulotomy:

a the laser is absorbed by the pigment in the eye

b it can elicit propionibacterium acne endophthalmitis

c raised intraocular pressure is higher in sulcus fixated lenses than 'in the bag' lenses

d complications of lens subluxation are most commonly seen with plate haptic lenses

e pupil block glaucoma is a complication.

152 In a patient with lattice dystrophy:

a the lesion usually involves the central cornea and spares the periphery

b the condition usually presents with recurrent erosion corneal syndrome

c the main type of amyloid is amyloid P

d presence of amyloid within the vitreous is common

e compared with macular or granular dystrophy, recurrence in the corneal graft is higher.

149

In accommodative esotropia, esotropia results from excessive accommodation in response to high hypermetropia. The age of onset is usually between 2 and 3 years of age. It is rarely detected before the age of 6 months. Cycloplegic refraction is essential as accommodation can underestimate the hypermetropia. Inferior oblique overaction and dissociated vertical deviation can occur in accommodative esotropia. Operating on the muscle does not resolve the esotropia as the eye will still converge when the eye attempts to accommodate.

150

β radiation has a deeper tissue penetration than α radiation. True exfoliation is a feature of infra-red radiation which is a form of non-ionising radiation. Dry eye and limbal stem cell failure occur with ionising radiation which can lead to corneal perforation. The lens is more vulnerable than the retina to radiation damage. Radiation retinopathy is the result of microangiopathy.

151

Nd:YAG laser works by breaking molecular bonds in tissue. Unlike argon laser, YAG laser is not absorbed by pigment. In a patient with sequestered focus of propriobacterium acne in the capsule, disruption of the capsule can give rise to endophthalmitis. Post-YAG capsulotomy-induced ocular hypertension is more common and is higher in patients with sulcus fixated lenses than those with 'in the bag' lenses. Lens subluxation is uncommon but can occur with plate haptic lens. Pupil block glaucoma can occur if there is prolapse of vitreous into the anterior chamber.

152

Lattice dystrophy is an autosomal dominant condition. The lesions typically involve the central cornea with clear intervening spaces. The periphery is spared. The condition usually presents as recurrent corneal erosion syndrome. Vision is usually normal until the 40s. The most common type of amyloid seen is amyloid P rather than amyloid A. Most cases of lattice dystrophy have amyloidosis confined to the cornea. It has a higher recurrent rate within the graft compared with other forms of stromal dystrophy.

153 True statements about latent nystagmus include:

a   it is more common than manifest latent nystagmus

b   it is absent when both eyes are open

c   the fast phase of the nystagmus is towards the occluded eye

d   in the presence of congenital esotropia, squint operation usually abolishes latent nystagmus

e   the amplitude decreases with age.

154 24 hours post-trabeculectomy:

a   a minus lens can usually improve the vision in patients with shallow anterior chamber

b   an increase in the intraocular pressure is usually caused by malignant glaucoma

c   the presence of choroidal effusion is associated with increased risk of trabeculectomy failure

d   shallow anterior chamber with iris-to-cornea touch does not require intervention

e   shallow anterior chamber with lens-to-cornea touch requires immediate reformation of the anterior chamber.

155 The following are true about chronic primary angle-closure glaucoma:

a   occurs most commonly in a hypermetropic patient

b   chronic retrobulbar pain is a feature

c   cataract extraction often decreases the pressure

d   laser iridotomy is not useful

e   progressive angle closure may occur in the presence of a patent peripheral iridectomy.

156 The following are true about gases used in retina surgery:

a   an ideal gas is one with low surface tension

b   expansion of gas is due to diffusion of oxygen and carbon dioxide

c   sulphur hexafluoride usually dissolves completely one week after injection

d   sulphur hexafluoride is more expansile than perfluoropropane

e   nuclear sclerosis is a complication of intravitreal gas usage.

153

Latent nystagmus is more often seen than manifest latent nystagmus. It is common in congenital esotropia. The nystagmus is absent with both eyes open and the fast phase of the nystagmus is towards the occluded eye. Surgery on the muscle does not abolish it. With time, the amplitude of the nystagmus decreases.

154

A shallow anterior chamber causes anterior movement of the lens, resulting in myopia. Malignant glaucoma is an uncommon cause of raised intraocular pressure even after trabeculectomy. One must exclude blockage of the sclerotomy by iris tissue, failure of filtration due to tight sutures or retained viscoelastic. Choroidal effusion is a common early finding following trabeculectomy and usually has no long-term implications. Shallow anterior chamber with iris-to-cornea touch is usually a transient phenomenon and needs only observation. Lens-to-cornea touch requires early reformation due to the risk of corneal decompensation and cataract.

155

Chronic angle-closure glaucoma can occur in patients with chronic open-angle glaucoma. It is more common in females and hypermetropic patients. Pain is not a feature. The angle closure can be abolished with cataract extraction provided there is no anterior synechiae. Laser iridotomy should be tried in these patients to break the pupillary block. Progressive angle closure may occur in the presence of a patent peripheral iridectomy and repeated periodic gonioscopy is imperative.

156

Intravitreal gases are used as volume replacement after vitrectomy and to retinal tamponade. The most commonly used gases are air, sulphur hexafluoride (SF6) and perfluoropropane (C3F8). Air dissolves most rapidly (5 days) followed by SF6 (2 weeks) and C3F8 (2 months). Expansion of gas is caused by diffusion of oxygen and carbon dioxide. Air does not expand, SF6 expands to twice its volume and C3F8 expands by about 4 times. Posterior subcapsular cataract is a complication of using intravitreal gas.

157 With regard to viscoelastic substances:

a   they have the ability to transform from gel into liquid under pressure

b   healon is a cohesive viscoelastic

c   a cohesive viscoelastic has better endothelial protective function

d   capsulorrhexis is easier to perform with a cohesive viscoelastic

e   a dispersive viscoelastic is easier to insert and remove.

158 Silicone oil:

a   is more effective than SF6 in the management of proliferative vitreoretinopathy

b   is lighter than water

c   causes abnormal ERG and EOG

d   acts as a plus lens in aphakic eyes

e   can be used instead of gas to avoid posturing.

159 Vitritis is a prominent feature in:

a   multiple choroiditis

b   acute multifocal placoid punctate epitheliopathy (AMPPE)

c   punctate inner choroidopathy

d   progressive outer retinal necrosis (PORN)

e   birdshot choroidopathy.

160 The advantages of indocyanine green (ICG) over fluorescein angiography (FFA) include:

a   better visualisation of retinal vasculature

b   better visualisation of the choroidal circulation

c   does not result in skin and urine discolouration

d   less nausea after injection

e   an exciting light source is not required.

157 (a) (b) (d)

Viscoelastics have pseudoplasticity properties, i.e. the ability to transform under pressure from gel to liquid. Viscoelastics can be divided into cohesive and dispersive types. Healon is a cohesive viscoelastic and viscoat is dispersive. A cohesive viscoelastic has better shock absorption, provides a better view for capsulorrhexis and is easier to insert and to remove.

A dispersive viscoelastic gives better coating and endothelial protection but gives a poorer view and is more difficult to insert and remove.

158 (b) (c) (d) (e)

Silicone oil is used as a long-lasting volume replacement following vitrectomy. It is more effective than SF6 in the management of proliferative vitreoretinopathy. It is lighter than water and very viscid. The use of silicone oil has been associated with abnormal ERG and EOG which may indicate a certain degree of retinal toxicity. In the aphakic eye, it acts as a plus lens and in the phakic eye as a minus lens. In those who cannot posture, such as the elderly, silicone oil can be used instead of gas.

159 (a) (b)

Vitritis is often minimal or absent in punctate inner choroidopathy, progressive outer retinal necrosis and birdshot choroidopathy.

160 (b) (c) (d)

ICG is highly protein bound and therefore does not leak out from the choroidal vasculature. This makes it ideal for the study of choroidal circulation and pathology. It is excreted unchanged by the liver and does not discolour skin or urine. Nausea is less common compared with FFA. ICG requires an exciting light source like FFA.

Quick fix

- Ultrasound travels slower in silicone oil (980m/sec) than in vitreous (1532m/sec).

- Biometry in an eye with silicone oil gives a falsely longer axial length.

161 True statements about par planitis include:

a   it is uncommon before the age of 10

b   multiple sclerosis is a common association

c   involvement of the anterior segment excludes this diagnosis

d   macular oedema is the most common cause of poor vision

e   systemic steroids are the treatment of choice for reducing inflammation.

162 Post-operatively, an eye has a refraction of +1.50D which was originally planned to be −0.50D. The following may be responsible:

a   nuclear sclerosis

b   asteroid hyalosis

c   little applanation during A-scan

d   posterior vitreous detachment

e   eccentric staphyloma.

163 Characteristics of toxoplasmosis include:

a   most cases of ocular toxoplasmosis result from ingestion of oocytes

b   siblings of patients with ocular toxoplasmosis rarely develop ocular findings

c   the organism typically involves the superficial retinal layer

d   serum Ig M anti-toxoplasma antibody is useful for the diagnosis of ocular toxoplasmosis

e   toxoplasma uveitis involving the posterior pole usually resolves spontaneously.

164 In biometry for intraocular lens calculation:

a   intraocular lens calculation using traditional keratometry in patients who have had photorefractive surgery will result in post-operative hypermetropia

b   videokeratography is more accurate than manual keratometry in patients who have had photorefractive surgery

c   error in keratometry measurement has a greater effect than axial length measurement

d   the velocity of ultrasound is faster in the silicone oil than in vitreous

e   axial length in a patient with silicone oil will give a falsely high value.

161 (d)

Par planitis is characterised by vitreous condensation and cellular aggregation in the inferior vitreous body. There are two peaks for its incidence: 5–15 and 25–35 years of age. It has no known cause.
In chronic cases, there may be a posterior subcapsular cataract, posterior synechiae and/or band keratopathy. The main cause of visual loss is macular oedema.
The treatment of choice for poor vision secondary to macular oedema is subtenon corticosteroid.

162 (c) (e)

A hypermetropic calculation will result if the axial length is falsely long and vice versa. Asteroid hyalosis and posterior vitreous detachment can give a shorter axial length than expected by reflecting the ultrasound before it reaches the retina.
Insufficient applanation can create a fluid space between the scan and the cornea, giving a falsely high axial length. Eccentric staphyloma also gives falsely long axial length if the ultrasound is not aimed at the macula. Nuclear sclerosis does not affect the biometry.

163 (b) (c) (e)

The majority of ocular toxoplasmosis is acquired through congenital transmission. Once immunity is established the subsequent foetuses are rarely infected. The organisms have a predilection for superficial retina. Serum Ig G anti-toxoplasma antibody is useful for the diagnosis. Reactivation of a toxoplasma lesion can give rise to self-limiting posterior uveitis; unless important structures or vision are threatened, treatment is not necessary.

164 (a) (b) (e)

Photorefractive surgery flattens the cornea and can result in miscalculation of intraocular lens power, giving a more hypermetropic calculation than expected. Videokeratography assesses more points on the cornea and provides more accurate keratometric results. In biometry, error in axial length measurement has a greater effect on the result than error in keratometric measurement. Ultrasonic waves travel more slowly in silicone oil and therefore give a falsely high axial length measurement.

165 The following are true about A pattern strabismus:

a the eye is less exotropic or more esotropic on up-gaze

b it is associated with overaction of the superior oblique muscle

c it is seen in Crouzon's disease

d it can be treated by anterio-posterior displacement of the inferior oblique muscle

e it can be treated by upward transposition of the medial rectus muscle.

166 With regard to medication used in cataract surgery:

a flurbiprofen can be used to prevent miosis but has no mydriatic effect

b intracameral lignocaine must be preservative-free

c the use of adrenaline in the infusion fluid is contraindicated because of the risk of cystoid macular oedema

d acetylcholine is used to constrict the pupil rapidly

e subconjunctival antibiotics have been shown to reduce the rate of post-operative endophthalmitis.

167 The following changes are responsible for involutional entropion:

a lateral canthal laxity

b orbital fat atrophy

c lower lid retractor laxity

d shallowing of the inferior fornix

e spasm of the orbicularis oculi.

168 In orbital myositis:

a an underlying cause can be found in the majority of patients

b the most commonly involved muscles are the superior and medial recti

c CT scan shows enlargement of the muscle belly with sparing of the tendon

d the pain is worse on looking away from the action of the affected muscle

e systemic non-steroidal anti-inflammatory drugs should be tried before systemic steroid.

165

A pattern strabismus occurs when the eye is less exotropic or more esotropic on up-gaze. It is associated with overaction of the superior oblique muscles. In craniosynostosis such as Crouzon's disease or Apert's syndrome, there is often inferior oblique overaction, giving rise to a V pattern. Inferior oblique muscle weakening does not improve the A pattern. Transposition of the horizontal recti can be used to reduce the A pattern – this is achieved by moving the medial rectus upwards or by moving the lateral rectus downwards.

166

Flurbiprofen can be used pre-operatively to prevent miosis but it has no intrinsic mydriatic effect. It can also be used to reduce inflammation if corticosteroids are contraindicated. Any drug used in the anterior chamber should be preservative-free because preservatives can damage the endothelium. Unpreserved adrenaline is added to the infusion solution to prevent miosis during phacoemulsification. Acetylcholine is used for rapid pupillary constriction. Although subconjunctival antibiotics are given routinely at the end of cataract surgery, studies have not shown a clear reduction of the endophthalmitis rate.

167

The following changes are believed to have contributed to involutional entropion:

- fat atrophy
- laxity of the medial and lateral canthal tendons
- laxity of the inferior retractor
- over-riding of the pre-tarsal muscle by the pre-septal muscle.

Shortening of the inferior fornix causes cicatricial entropion, and spasm of the orbicularis oculi causes spastic entropion.

168

Orbital myositis is idiopathic in the majority of patients. It is part of the spectrum of idiopathic orbital inflammatory syndrome. The superior and medial recti are most commonly involved. CT scan shows enlargement of the muscle belly with involvement of the tendon. Pain is worse when the eye looks away from the action of the affected muscle. Forced duction test is often positive. Chronic cases can lead to fibrosis and restriction of ocular movement. In the acute stage, a non-steroidal anti-inflammatory drug may be sufficient to control the inflammation. If this fails, systemic steroids are usually required.

169 Heterochromic iridis occurs in the following:

a   acquired Horner's syndrome

b   Sturge-Weber's syndrome

c   Waardenburg's syndrome

d   Hirschprung's disease

e   naevus of Ota.

170 Latanoprost:

a   decreases the formation of aqueous humour

b   should be avoided in the presence of anterior uveitis

c   causes iris hyperpigmentation by inciting melanocyte hyperplasia

d   should be avoided in pseudophakic patients

e   anti-glaucoma effect is reduced with the concurrent use of a non-steroidal anti-inflammatory drug.

171 In nanophthalmos:

a   the palpebral fissure is reduced

b   intraocular structures are disorganised

c   microspherophakia is usual

d   the sclera is abnormally thickened

e   intraocular surgery is associated with rhegmatogenous retinal detachment.

172 Regarding Sturge-Weber's syndrome:

a   the port-wine stain does not cross the midline

b   glaucoma is more common in a patient with upper lid rather than lower lid involvement

c   recurrent epilepsy and mental retardation are features

d   tram-line appearance on the plain skull X-ray is the result of calcification of the abnormal cerebral vessel

e   expulsive haemorrhage is a recognised risk during cataract surgery.

169

Congenital rather than acquired Horner's syndrome is associated with heterochromia iridis with the affected side being lighter. Sympathetic innervation is important for the migration of melanocytes into the iris. Sturge-Weber's syndrome can give rise to ipsilateral iris hyperpigmentation. Waardenburg's syndrome causes hypochromia of the iris. Hirschprung's disease results from abnormal sympathetic nervous system development and hence abnormal melanocyte migration. Naevus of Ota causes increased pigmentation of the affected side.

170

Latanoprost works by increasing uveoscleral outflow. It causes blood aqueous barrier instability and should be avoided in anterior uveitis. It should also be avoided in aphakic and pseudophakic patients due to the risk of cystoid macular oedema. Iris hyperpigmentation results from increased production of melanin by the melanocytes. Non-steroidal anti-inflammatory drugs which inhibit the formation of prostaglandins have no effect on latanoprost, which is a prostaglandin analogue.

171

In nanophthalmos, the axial length of the eye is reduced. The lens, however, is of normal size and this increases the risk of pupillary block. The sclera is abnormally thickened and this is thought to cause uveal effusion syndrome and rhegmatogenous retinal detachment, especially after intraocular surgery, through vortex vein compression.

172

Sturge-Weber's syndrome is a type of phakomatoses. It has a sporadic occurrence. The condition is characterised by a port-wine stain involving the trigeminal distribution. However, the lesion often crosses the midline. Glaucoma is a common complication due to increased episcleral venous pressure, and is more common if the port-wine stain involves the upper lid. Recurrent epilepsy and mental retardation occur in about 50% of cases. Cerebral angiomatosis causes cerebral calcification in a tram-line fashion. Diffuse choroidal haemangioma is common and increases the risk of expulsive haemorrhage during intraocular surgery.

173 The pairing of the following are correct:

a epiblepharon – punctate keratitis

b dermatochalasis – superior visual field defect

c blepharochalasis – allergic dermatitis

d floppy eyelid syndrome – chronic papillary conjunctivitis

e brow ptosis – facial nerve palsy.

174 A patient with an orbital implant develops a superior sulcus deformity. The following methods are useful in correcting or reducing the deformity:

a levator resection

b increasing the size of the orbital implant

c lower lid tightening

d placement of cartilage along the orbital floor

e mucous membrane graft.

175 In Tolosa-Hunt's syndrome:

a the lesion is located at the orbital apex

b the cause is usually a metastatic tumour

c visual loss is common

d orbital inflammation is often absent

e systemic steroids usually relieve the pain before ophthalmoplegia.

176 Regarding systemic lupus erythematosus (SLE):

a the diagnosis is made by the presence of characteristic anti-nuclear antibodies

b the majority of patients are female of child-bearing age

c superficial punctate keratitis is the most common cornea pathology associated with SLE

d cotton wool spots are a feature of SLE retinopathy

e cerebrovascular accident is the main cause of death.

173

In epiblepharon there is excess pre-tarsal skin and orbicularis oculi. This can cause misdirection of the eyelashes, resulting in corneal irritation and punctate keratitis. Dermatochalasis is seen in the elderly due to excess upper lid skin. Overhanging of the skin can cause superior visual field defects. Blepharochalasis affects younger people with recurrent inflammation and swelling of the upper lid. This can lead to loosening of the skin and levator dehiscence. It is not caused by allergy. Floppy eyelid syndrome typically affects middle-aged overweight males. The upper lid everts easily during sleep, causing mechanical irritation. Chronic papillary conjunctivitis and punctate keratitis are common. Brow ptosis can be involutional or the result of facial nerve palsy.

174

Loss of volume or shifting of the orbital implant usually causes a superior sulcus deformity in an eye with an orbital implant. Increasing the size of the orbital implant is useful. If the lower lid is lax, tightening the lid will allow the prosthesis to be placed more superiorly and reduces the deformity. Placing cartilage in the orbital floor will help to elevate the implant and reduces the deformity.

175

Tolosa-Hunt's syndrome involves the cavernous sinus. It is thought to be an extra-orbital idiopathic inflammatory disorder. There is pain and ophthalmoplegia due to involvement of the third, fourth and sixth cranial nerves. It is a diagnosis of exclusion. As the optic nerve does not enter the cavernous sinus, visual involvement is rare. Proptosis is minimal and orbital inflammation is often absent. Systemic steroid is the treatment of choice. Pain usually responds to treatment first before ophthalmoplegia.

176

Systemic lupus erythematosus is a systemic collagen vascular disease. The underlying pathogenesis is caused by autoimmune necrotising vasculitis. The majority of patients are female and of child-bearing age. Diagnosis is made clinically by the presence of specific signs. Superficial punctate keratitis is the most common sign in the cornea. Cotton wool spots are characteristic of SLE retinopathy. Proliferative retinopathy can occur but is uncommon. The main cause of death is renal failure.

177 The following B scan ultrasound features favour a diagnosis of choroidal detachment rather than retinal detachment:

a   dome-shaped elevation

b   presence of fluid level

c   attachment of vortex veins to the elevated area

d   attachment of the elevation to the optic disc

e   vitreous opacities.

178 The following genetic disorders are associated with the development of multiple basal cell carcinoma:

a   Gorlin's syndrome

b   xeroderma pigmentosa

c   incontinentia pigmenti

d   albinism

e   neurofibromatosis.

179 The pairings of the following concerning glaucoma are true:

a   Scheie's procedure – removal of full-thickness sclera

b   trabeculectomy – partial removal of the ciliary body

c   goniotomy – incision of trabecular meshwork

d   trabeculotomy – partial removal of trabecular meshwork

e   trabeculodialysis – creation of a cyclodialysis cleft.

177

Choroidal detachment tends to have a smooth and dome-shaped outline. Fluid level is common and the vortex vein may be seen attached to the elevation.

178

Gorlin's syndrome is also called the naevoid basal cell carcinoma syndrome. It is an autosomal dominant disorder characterised by development of multiple basal cell carcinoma in early life. Xeroderma pigmentosa is an autosomal recessive disorder. The DNA repair mechanism is defective, resulting in an increased incidence of skin tumours upon exposure to ultraviolet light. Albinism lacks melanin which is protective against ultraviolet light. As a result, the skin is at risk of various tumours including basal cell carcinoma. Incontinentia pigmenti is an X-linked dominant disorder. The patient develops erythema and bullae on the skin and proliferative retinopathy. The risk of developing basal cell carcinoma is not increased. Neurofibromatosis does not cause an increased incidence of basal cell carcinoma.

179

Scheie's procedure creates a full-thickness sclerotomy. Hence, intraocular pressure is less controlled and hypotony is common. Trabeculectomy involves removing part of the sclera to create a sclerotomy which is then covered by a scleral flap. The procedure is performed anterior to the ciliary body. Goniotomy is performed in congenital glaucoma to create a communication between the anterior chamber and Schlemm's canal. It involves incision of the trabecular meshwork at a point between Schwalbe's line and the scleral spur. Trabeculotomy establishes a communication between the anterior chamber and Schlemm's canal by partial removal of the trabecular meshwork (goniotomy *ab externo*). Trabeculodialysis involves incision of Schwalbe's line followed by disinsertion of the trabecular meshwork from the scleral spur.

180 Features of primary congenital glaucoma include the following:

a   males are more commonly affected than females

b   siblings have a 5% chance of being affected

c   there is enlargement of both the cornea and the axial length

d   Haab's striae is caused by tears in Descemet's membrane

e   the amount of optic disc cupping can be used to predict visual prognosis.

181 The following drugs are known to cause anterior uveitis:

a   rifabutin

b   streptokinase

c   quinidine

d   cidofovir

e   metipranolol.

182 The following are true concerning optic nerve trauma in head injuries:

a   it usually involves the intracranial portion of the optic nerve

b   an altitudinal visual field defect is common

c   optic atrophy is a common complication

d   delay latency in the visual evoked potential may occur

e   it usually responds to optic nerve fenestration.

183 With regard to AC/A (accommodative convergence/ accommodation) ratio:

a   it refers to the amount of accommodative convergence in prism dioptres per unit of accommodation

b   it decreases with age

c   it is reduced with phopholine iodide

d   it decreases in exotropia

e   it is better measured with the heterophoria rather than the gradient method.

180 (a) (b) (c) (d)

Primary congenital glaucoma affects males more often than females. About 60 to 80% of cases have bilateral involvement. The inheritance is multifactorial; siblings and offspring have a 5% chance of acquiring the disease. The raised intraocular pressure causes global enlargement of the eye. Haab's striae results from tears in Descemet's membrane. Optic disc cupping develops early but usually reverses with treatment of the intraocular pressure. Corneal opacities and refractive amblyopia usually cause poor vision.

181 (a) (b) (c) (d) (e)

Other drugs that have been reported to cause uveitis include oral contraceptives, hepatitis B and BCG vaccines, interleukin-3, interleukin-6, diethylcarbamazine and disodium pamidronate.

182 (c) (d)

Optic nerve trauma in head injuries often occurs in the intracanalicular portion. The visual field defect is usually a central scotoma. Optic atrophy is common and the visual evoked potential will show a delayed latency. Optic nerve fenestration is usually performed in patients with optic nerve sheath haematoma – however, in most traumatic optic neuropathies the optic nerve appears normal on CT or MRI scan, and optic nerve fenestration is of uncertain benefit in such cases.

183 (a) (c)

AC/A ratio refers to the amount of accommodative convergence needed in prism dioptre per unit dioptre of accommodation. This ratio tends to remain unchanged throughout life. Phopholine iodide stimulates accommodation and therefore may reduce the ratio. AC/A ratio is increased in exotropia. AC/A ratio can be measured with either the gradient or heterophoria method but the former is more accurate.

184 The female carrier of the following X-linked conditions may show fundal changes:

a   choroideremia

b   retinoschisis

c   ocular albinism

d   retinitis pigmentosa

e   Norrie's disease.

185 Features of cluster headaches include:

a   greater predilection in males than females

b   the pupil is typically enlarged during the attack

c   ptosis is a feature

d   prodromal visual symptoms are typical

e   rhinorrhoea is common.

186 Mooren's ulcer:

a   has a better prognosis if the patient is less than 40 years of age

b   tends to affect both eyes in older patients

c   is associated with Wegener's granulomatosis in 20% of cases

d   is usually associated with scleritis

e   may be treated with limbal conjunctival excision.

187 Advantages of fornix-based over limbal-based conjunctival flaps during trabeculectomy include:

a   better surgical exposure

b   less post-operative wound leakage

c   easier wound closure

d   formation of a more diffuse bleb

e   better long-term intraocular pressure control.

184

In choroideremia, ocular albinism and retinitis pigmentosa, pigmentary changes may be observed in the peripheral retina of the female carrier. Retinoschisis and Norrie's disease are not associated with abnormal retinal findings in the female carriers.

185

Cluster headaches occur more commonly in males than females. The pain is severe and confined to within the region of the eye. During the attacks, conjunctival redness, lacrimation and Horner's syndrome can occur. Other features include orbital swelling, rhinorrhea and nasal congestion. Unlike migraine, prodromal visual symptoms are uncommon.

186

Mooren's ulcer is a peripheral ulcerative keratitis that begins in the corneoscleral limbus and progresses centrally and circumferentially. The condition is idiopathic and not associated with scleritis. In the elderly, the disease tends to be unilateral and associated with good prognosis. In the young, especially in people of African origin, the disease tends to be bilateral and more aggressive. Excision of the limbal conjunctival may be useful in some cases. Other treatment options include systemic steroids and immunosuppression.

187

The advantages of fornix-based over limbal-based conjunctival flaps during trabeculectomy include: better surgical exposure, easier wound closure and formation of a more diffuse bleb. Post-operative wound leakage is more common in fornix-based flaps compared with limbal-based flaps. The long-term intraocular pressure control is equivocal in either approach.

188 The following features on B scan suggest a rhegmatogenous retinal detachment:

a absence of echogenicity behind the membrane

b attachment of the membrane to the optic disc

c full mobility of the membrane

d high echogenicity of the membrane

e attachment of the membrane to multiple sites away from the disc.

189 Iridoschisis:

a usually involves the inferior quadrant of the iris

b results from a split between the iris stroma and the pigment epithelium

c can be caused by mydriatics

d is associated with glaucoma in 50% of cases

e can cause endothelial decompensation.

190 Riley-Day's syndrome:

a is an autosomal recessive disorder

b causes corneal anaesthesia

c results in a decrease in lacrimation

d causes decreased sweating

e may be associated with an increased urine HVA (homovanillic acid).

191 In marginal keratitis:

a the lesion is typically found where the cornea rests against the eyelid

b there is a clear area between the lesion and the limbus

c cornea scrape usually yields Gram-positive bacteria

d lid swab usually yields *Streptococcus*

e systemic tetracycline can be used to prevent recurrence.

188

Rhegmatogenous retinal membranes are not associated with fluid behind the membrane. A fully mobile membrane suggests a posterior vitreous detachment. The membrane has the same echogenicity as the retina. Presence of multiple sites of attachment is suggestive of tractional retinal detachment.

189

Iridoschisis is a degenerative disorder involving the lower quadrant of the iris near the pupil. It is an uncommon condition and usually affects the elderly. The splitting of the iris occurs between the anterior and the posterior stroma. It is idiopathic in most cases but acute angle-closure glaucoma and use of miotics such as pilocarpine are contributing factors. It is associated with glaucoma in 50% of cases and may lead to endothelial decompensation.

190

Riley-Day's syndrome or familial dysautonomia is a rare autosomal recessive disorder characterised by an abnormal autonomic nervous system and sensory function. There is a deficiency of the enzyme dopamine β-hydroxylase. This causes an increased urinary HVA (homovanillic acid). The ophthalmic features include corneal anaesthesia, decreased lacrimation, anisocoria and ptosis. Systemic features include paroxysmal hypertension, increased sweating and emotional lability.

191

Marginal keratitis is an immune disorder caused by hypersensitivity to the staphylococcal toxin. Blepharitis is common. The lesion is characterised by infiltrate with a clear zone between the lesion and the limbus. The lesion is usually localised to the area of the cornea which is in close contact with the eyelid. Lid swabs usually reveal *Staphylococcus aureus* but the cornea scrap is sterile. Treatment consists of weak steroids. Lid hygiene and tetracycline can rid the lids of *Staphylococcus* and prevent recurrence.

192 In a patient with suspected fungal keratitis, the following stains can be used for identification:

a   haematoxylin and eosin (H&E)

b   periodic acid schiff (PAS)

c   methenamine silver

d   calcofluor white

e   Giemsa stain.

193 In a pleomorphic adenoma of the lacrimal gland:

a   the globe is usually displaced inferomedially

b   the tumour contains ductules of the epithelial cells and fatty tissue

c   pain is uncommon

d   CT scan usually reveals an increase in orbital volume

e   biopsy of the lesion is recommended to exclude malignancy.

194 Posterior polar cataract:

a   is usually a congenital disorder

b   involves the cortex and the capsule

c   causes more visual symptoms than an anterior polar cataract

d   is associated with a higher incidence of posterior capsule rupture during cataract surgery

e   is associated with phacodonesis.

195 In aqueous tear deficiency:

a   there is a reduction in the tear meniscus

b   facial nerve palsy may be a cause

c   inferior punctate keratopathy is a feature

d   antihistamine reduces aqueous tear production

e   tear break up time is decreased.

192

The cell wall of the fungus can be identified using PAS, methenamine silver, calcofluor white and Giemsa stain. Calcofluor white also stains acanthamoeba and Giemsa also stains chlamydia.

193

Pleomorphic adenoma is a benign tumour of the lacrimal gland composed of ductules of the epithelial cells and fibrous myxoid stroma. It grows slowly, causing downward and medial displacement of the globe. Orbital bone erosion without destruction is common, resulting in expansion of the orbital volume. Pain is rare unless the tumour undergoes malignant transformation. The treatment of choice is excision without biopsy because of the risk of orbital seeding leading to recurrence and, rarely, malignant transformation.

194

Posterior polar cataracts involve the cortex and the capsule. It is a congenital disorder and can be sporadic or familial. Visual symptoms are usually more common than anterior polar cataracts because of their location and also their tendency to progress. Posterior capsule rupture is a common complication during cataract surgery. Zonular dialysis is not a feature.

195

In aqueous tear deficiency, the tear meniscus is reduced and there may be punctate keratopathy of the inferior paracentral region. Facial nerve palsy affects the parasympathetic supply to the lacrimal gland and reduces tear production. Antihistamines, oral contraceptives and atropine can cause dry eyes by reducing aqueous tear production. The tear break up time is usually normal in aqueous tear deficiency.

196 In pellucid marginal degeneration:

a   the peripheral inferior cornea is thinned and flattened

b   with-the-rule astigmatism is common

c   Munson's sign is a feature

d   Fleischer's ring is commonly seen

e   wedge resection can improve vision.

197 In the Herpetic Eye Disease Study:

a   oral acyclovir is effective in preventing recurrence of herpetic keratitis

b   oral acyclovir is not effective in preventing uveitis

c   oral acyclovir is effective in preventing stromal keratitis

d   topical acyclovir is effective in preventing stromal keratitis

e   topical corticosteroids are safe and effective in stromal keratitis.

198 During retinal detachment, the following conditions favour the use of an encircling scleral buckle:

a   posterior breaks

b   U-shaped tear with 'fish-mouthing'

c   extensive retinal detachment without detectable breaks

d   aphakic retinal detachment

e   lattice degeneration in three or more quadrants.

199 In Brown's syndrome, the following features are observed:

a   hypotropia of the affected eye

b   poor elevation in abduction

c   V pattern

d   downshoot in adduction

e   widening of the palpebral fissure in adduction.

196

Pellucid marginal degeneration is an ectatic condition characterised by thinning and flattening of the peripheral inferior cornea. This gives rise to against-the-rule astigmatism. Munson's sign is a non-specific sign and can occur in any condition which causes protrusion of the cornea. Unlike keratoconus, Fleischer's ring and Vogt's striae are not seen. Wedge resection of the thinned area can improve vision.

197

Oral acyclovir is effective in preventing the recurrence of herpetic keratitis and uveitis but not stromal keratitis. Topical corticosteroids are safe and effective in stromal keratitis.

198

A radial scleral buckle is preferable in patients with posterior breaks or large U-shaped tears to prevent 'fish-mouthing'. Other indications for encirclage include: multiple breaks in three or more quadrants, mild proliferative vitreoretinopathy, excessive drainage or subretinal fluid.

199

Brown's syndrome is characterised by defective elevation in adduction. The affected eye may be hypotropic in the primary position. Other features include: V pattern, downshoot in adduction, positive forced duction test and widening of the palpebral fissure in adduction.

Quick fix

- Herpetic eye disease studies showed that oral acyclovir does not have added benefit to herpetic keratitis if the patient is already on topical treatment.

- Treatment with oral acyclovir during acute herpetic epithelial keratitis does not prevent the development of stromal keratitis.

- Oral acyclovir following an acute attack of herpetic stromal keratitis may reduce the rate of recurrence.

- Topical steroid is useful in speeding up the recovery of herpetic stromal keratitis.

200 A 40-year-old patient presents with a 4-week history of persistent right red eye despite using chloramphenicol eye drops for the past 3 weeks. Further examination may reveal the following:

a   history of facial trauma

b   delayed fluorescence disappearance test

c   history of non-specific urethritis

d   positive conjunctival swab for *Haemophilus* species

e   acne rosacea.

201 The following are true about candida endophthalmitis:

a   it occurs exclusively in immunocompromised patients

b   retinal infiltrates may give rise to Roth spots

c   a 'string of pearls' appearance occurs with retinal infiltrates

d   intravenous fluconazole is the preferred treatment rather than amphotericin B

e   intravitreal amphotericin B is more effective than intravenous amphotericin B.

202 In cystoid macular oedema following cataract surgery:

a   the cause is an increased permeability of the perifoveal capillaries

b   the majority of patients are asymptomatic

c   a common presentation is poor vision 1 week after cataract extraction

d   chronic cystoid macular oedema does not respond to treatment

e   macular grid laser is effective.

203 The findings of the United Kingdom Prospective Diabetes Study (UKPDS) include:

a   an improved glucose control reduces the risk of developing retinopathy in type II diabetes

b   intensive glucose control with either insulin or oral hypoglycaemic drugs can reduce microvascular complications

c   a decrease in the glycosylated haemoglobin concentration reduces the risk of microvascular complications

d   tight control of hypertension reduces microvascular complications

e   an angiotensin-converting enzyme (ACE) inhibitor is better than a β-blocker in preventing macrovascular complications.

200

This patient has a chronic conjunctivitis defined as the presence of conjunctivitis for more than 1 week despite treatment. Blockage of the nasolacrimal duct can cause chronic conjunctivitis. Therefore, a history of facial trauma and delayed fluorescence disappearance test are relevant. Non-specific urethritis may be caused by chlamydia which in turn is a cause of chronic follicular conjunctivitis. Acne rosacea is associated with posterior blepharitis which may lead to chronic conjunctivitis. *Haemophilus* species can cause acute bacterial conjunctivitis which responds to chloramphenicol.

201

Candida endophthalmitis occurs in disseminated candidiasis and can occur in immunocompetent patients such as intravenous drug users. The lesion usually begins in the subretinal areas and extends into the retina and the vitreous. Roth spots can occur with retinal infiltrates. Vitreous infiltrate can give rise to a 'string of pearls' appearance. Amphotericin B is highly protein bound and therefore penetrates ocular tissue poorly. Systemic fluconazole is the treatment of choice for ocular endophthalmitis. In severe cases, vitrectomy and intravitreal amphotericin B are effective.

202

Cystoid macular oedema (CMO) following cataract surgery is caused by increased perifoveal capillary permeability. Fluorescein angiography shows the condition to be common but clinically most patients are asymptomatic. CMO typically occurs 2–6 months after cataract surgery. It is more common in the presence of complications such as a ruptured posterior capsule, lens malposition and chronic uveitis. Topical adrenaline and latanoprost also increase the incidence.
In patients with chronic CMO associated with lens malposition or adherence of vitreous to the wound, lens repositioning or exchange and vitrectomy can result in resolution of the oedema. Macular grid laser has not been shown to be effective.

203

The UKPDS is a randomised, prospective clinical trial of type II diabetes. The study shows that intensive control of blood glucose with either insulin or oral hypoglycaemic drugs slows down the progression of retinopathy and other microvascular complications of diabetes. Intensive blood pressure control slows down the progression of retinopathy and reduces the risk of both microvascular and macrovascular complications of diabetes. There are no clinical differences between ACE inhibitors and β-blockers

204 AMPPE (acute multifocal placoid pigment epitheliopathy):

a   is usually a bilateral condition

b   affects young males more commonly than females

c   is a self-limiting condition

d   shows hypofluorescence in the early phase of fluorescein angiography

e   shows reduced ERG and EOG recordings.

205 Pavingstone retinal degeneration:

a   is present in 50% of people over the age of 20

b   represents areas of ischaemic outer retina

c   is found mainly in the superior quadrants

d   does not predispose to retinal breaks

e   coalesces and gives rise to retinoschisis.

206 Disc drusen:

a   are of similar histology to retinal drusen

b   become progressively embedded with age

c   are associated with peripapillary haemorrhage

d   are associated with angioid streaks

e   are associated with retinitis pigmentosa.

207 Plus disease in retinopathy or prematurity is characterised by:

a   vitreous haze

b   lens opacities

c   pupillary rigidity

d   corneal haze

e   tortuosity of retinal vessels.

204

First described by Gass in 1968, acute posterior multifocal placoid pigment epitheliopathy (APMPPE) is an acquired inflammatory disorder affecting the retina, retinal pigment epithelium and choroid of otherwise young healthy adults, with equal male to female incidence. The disease is self-limited and is characterised by multiple yellowish-white placoid subretinal lesions of the posterior pole. The lesions are frequently bilateral and in various stages of evolution, typically resolving in weeks to months and leaving circumscribed areas of retinal pigment epithelial disturbance. Fluorescein angiography shows hypofluorescence in the early phase and this is either the result of blockage by the RPE or choroidal ischaemia. Electrophysiology tests show reduced ERG and EOG recordings.

205

Pavingstone retinal degeneration represents discrete areas of ischaemia involving the outer retina. It is seen in 22% of patients over the age of 20. It is most commonly located in the inferior retinal quadrant anterior to the equator. It does not give rise to retinal breaks. Retinoschisis is caused by coalescence of peripheral cystoid degeneration.

206

Disc drusen are of different composition to retinal drusen. With age, the drusen become exposed. They are associated with peripapillary subretinal neovascular membrane formation, angioid streaks and retinitis pigmentosa.

207

Plus disease implies dilation and tortuosity of the blood vessels near the optic nerve. It also includes the growth and dilation of abnormal blood vessels on the surface of the iris, rigidity of the pupil and vitreous haze. The diagnosis of plus disease is usually based on the appearance of the vessels near the optic nerve, as compared with standard retinal photographs. The presence of plus disease suggests a more fulminant or rapidly progressive course.

208 Common ocular findings in Goldenhar's syndrome include:

a hypertelorism

b eyelid coloboma

c optic disc coloboma

d microphthalmos

e decreased corneal sensation.

209 The following features distinguish optic disc swelling from papilloedema:

a the presence of relative afferent pupillary defect

b normal visual acuity

c absence of venous pulsation

d leakage of fluorescein from the optic nerve head during fluorescein angiography

e an enlarged blind spot.

210 In vernal keratoconjunctivitis:

a the condition is more common in cold than warm climates

b cobblestone appearance of the conjunctiva is seen almost exclusively in the upper tarsal conjunctiva

c interpalpebral corneal staining is a feature

d a shield ulcer seen in the superior cornea is always surrounded by infiltrates

e eye rubbing increases the severity of symptoms.

211 The following are indications for temporal clear corneal incision under local anaesthesia:

a an unco-operative patient

b deep sulcus

c presence of a superior filtering bleb

d with-the-rule astigmatism

e small pupil.

208

Goldenhar's syndrome is also called oculoauriculovertebral dysplasia. Eye signs include limbal dermoid, lid coloboma and microphthalmos.

209

Optic disc swelling causes abnormal optic nerve function with a relative afferent pupillary defect, colour desaturation and decreased visual acuity. Absence of venous pulsation, an enlarged blind spot and leakage of fluorescein from the optic nerve head occur in both optic disc swelling and papilloedema.

Quick fix

- Astigmatism following cataract surgery may be reduced by the following methods:
  - limbal incision
  - temporal approach
  - smaller incision.
- Indication for astigmatic keratotomy should be based on corneal astigmatism and not total astigmatism because of the contribution of lenticular astigmatism in the latter.

210

Vernal keratoconjunctivitis is more common in warm than cold climates. It is characterised by the presence of conjunctival cobblestones confined almost exclusively to the superior tarsal conjunctiva. Interpalebral corneal staining is a feature of dry eye. Shield ulcers are not associated with corneal infiltration. Eye rubbing can increase the discharge of mast cell mediators and increase the severity of symptoms.

211

The advantages of a temporal clear corneal incision include less astigmatic changes because the horizontal corneal diameter is longer than the vertical diameter. In addition, it allows easy access to the eye in patients with sunken globes. A superior filtering bleb may be compromised if the phacoemulsification is performed through a superior corneal incision. An unco-operative patient should have general anaesthesia. A temporal incision will worsen with-the-rule astigmatism. The location of the incision site does not affect pupil size.

212 With regard to cataract surgery in a patient with diabetes mellitus:

a progression of non-proliferative diabetic retinopathy in the operated eye is a feature

b progression of non-proliferative diabetic retinopathy in the non-operated eye is a feature

c progression of non-proliferative diabetic retinopathy is more common in women than men

d a small capsulorrhexis is preferable to avoid extrusion of the implant

e an implant with a large optic is preferable.

213 The following techniques are useful in repairing a large lower lid defect involving the margin following excision of basal cell carcinoma:

a Cutler-Beard's procedure

b Tenzel flap

c Hughes' procedure

d Mustarde rotation flap

e glabellar flap.

214 Meningioma of the orbit:

a results from intracranial extension in 90% of cases

b occurs more commonly in females than males

c is associated with neurofibromatosis type I

d is more often benign in children than adults

e can be treated with chemotherapy.

215 In a 6-month-old child with poor vision, myopic refraction is seen in:

a gyrate atrophy

b Leber's congenital amaurosis

c X-linked congenital stationary blindness

d blue cone monochromatism

e Norrie's disease.

212

Diabetes mellitus is associated with progression of non-proliferative diabetic retinopathy in the operated eye following cataract surgery. This progression is more common in women, in particular those who are overweight. A large capsulorrhexis and an implant with a large optic are preferable as this would allow better visualisation of the periphery and facilitate pan-photocoagulation.

213

Cutler-Beard's procedure is used in the repair of upper lid defect.
A glabellar flap is used for the repair of medial canthal skin defects.

Quick fix

- Full-thickness eyelid defects of extent up to 25% may be closed directly.

- Defects of extent 25% to 66% require cantholysis for closure without undue tension.

- Full-thickness eyelid defects of extent more than 66% require the use of flaps for satisfactory closure.

214

Only 10% of orbital meningiomas arise within the orbit, the rest result from intracranial extension, usually from the sphenoid bone or the olfactory groove. It is more common in females than males and is associated with neurofibromatosis type I. In children, orbital meningioma tends to be more aggressive with a propensity for intracranial spread. Well-circumscribed meningioma can be excised and the diffuse form treated with radiotherapy. Chemotherapy is not useful.

215

Gyrate atrophy is associated with myopia but the vision is not affected until adulthood. Leber's congenital amaurosis is associated with hypermetropic refraction. Myopic shift is a feature of X-linked congenital stationary blindness and blue cone monochromatism.

216 Features of de Morsier's syndrome include:

a   optic nerve hypoplasia

b   nystagmus

c   growth failure

d   absent septum callosum

e   basal encephalocele.

217 The effects of pregnancy include:

a   enlargement of uveal melanoma

b   progression of Grave's disease

c   reduction in the size of prolactinoma

d   increased incidence of diabetic macular oedema

e   enlargement of meningioma.

218 Diabetic papillopathy:

a   results from intracranial hypertension

b   is a feature of poor diabetic control

c   is associated with optic disc neovascularisation

d   usually resolves with laser photocoagulation

e   indicates poor visual prognosis.

219 In superior oblique myokymia:

a   there is repetitive large oscillation of the affected eye

b   ocular oscillation can be heard with a stethoscope

c   the oscillation is usually precipitated by reading

d   there is an association with cerebellar lesion

e   carbamazepine is useful.

216

de Morsier's syndrome or septo-optic dysplasia consists of a triad of optic nerve hypoplasia, nystagmus and growth failure. Neuro-imaging typically shows an absent septum pellucidum and basal encephalocele.

217

During pregnancy, uveal melanoma, prolactinoma and meningioma can undergo enlargement. Grave's disease becomes more severe. Diabetic retinopathy of any type tends to progress during pregnancy.

Quick fix

Chemicals and drugs that may cause optic neuropathy include:

- alcohol
- amiodarone
- chloramphenicol
- chlorpropamide
- digitalis
- ethambutol
- isoniazide
- methanol
- streptomycin.

218 **None**

Diabetic papillopathy is an uncommon complication of diabetes mellitus. It can occur in young or old patients and in type I or type II diabetes. There is no intracranial hypertension, the swelling may be unilateral or bilateral. Poor diabetic control is not a feature and laser photocoagulation does not help. The swelling may be the result of optic nerve head ischaemia, and telangiectasia may be seen, which can be confused with neovascularisation. The swelling usually resolves spontaneously and the vision is not affected.

219

Superior oblique myokymia is a rare disorder characterised by repetitive small amplitude oscillation of the globe. This oscillation may be vertical or oblique. The patient usually complains of diplopia, blurred vision or oscillopsia. The oscillation is best observed with a slit-lamp and can be heard with a stethoscope. It is often precipitated by reading. The condition is benign and a central nervous disorder is uncommon. Carbamazepine can reduce the oscillation.

220 The pairing of the following are correct:

a   opsoclonus – pituitary lesion

b   ocular bobbing – coma

c   ocular flutter – cerebellar lesion

d   ocular myoclonus – pontine stroke

e   spasmus nutan – neuroblastoma.

221 In a patient with a choroidal melanoma, the risk of metastasis is increased in the presence of:

a   epithelioid cell type

b   an anterior location

c   involvement of the vortex vein

d   the tumour extending through the Bruch's membrane

e   a large tumour.

222 Proliferative vitreoretinopathy:

a   results from proliferation of retinal pigment epithelial cells

b   is more common in younger patients

c   is increased in the presence of vitreous haemorrhage

d   is more common in retinal detachment treated with a scleral buckle compared with a vitrectomy

e   can be prevented with systemic steroid.

223 Features of multiple evanescent white dot syndrome include the following:

a   female predilection

b   presence of an enlarged blind spot despite a normal optic disc

c   vitritis being a prominent feature

d   fluorescein angiography shows early hyperfluorescence of the white lesions

e   electrophysiology studies indicate dysfunction of the inner retinal layer.

220

Opsoclonus is characterised by spontaneous chaotic rapid conjugate bursts of ocular saccades in all directions. In children it may be associated with neuroblastoma. Other associations include occult visceral carcinoma in adults and post-viral encephalitis. Ocular bobbing is characterised by fast downward ocular movements followed by a slow return of the eyes to the primary position. It is seen in comatose patients with major intracranial haemorrhage. Ocular flutter involves to-and-fro horizontal oscillations that occur when the patient attempts to fixate on a target in the primary position. It is associated with cerebellar lesion. Ocular myoclonus initially resembles ocular bobbing and then becomes more pendular. It is seen in patients with pontine stroke. Spasmus nutan is made up of a triad of nystagmus, involuntary head movement and an abnormal head posture. It usually resolves spontaneously and has no underlying cause.

221

The risk of metastasis in choroidal melanoma is increased in the presence of a large tumour, an anterior location of the tumour, a tumour composed mainly of epithelioid cells and involvement of the vortex vein. Extension of the tumour through Bruch's membrane is not associated with metastasis.

222

Proliferative vitreoretinopathy is a late complication of retinal surgery. It is caused by proliferation of retinal pigment epithelial cells on the retina. It is associated with vitreous haemorrhage and vitreous surgery. Conditions that release retinal pigment epithelial cells into the vitreous increase the risk of proliferative vitreoretinopathy, and include multiple or large breaks and the use of cryopexy.

223

Multiple evanescent white dot syndrome is often a unilateral condition affecting young female patients. The presentation is usually decreased vision with multiple white dots in the retinal pigment epithelium layer. An enlarged blind spot is common despite a normal optic disc. Vitritis is usually mild. Fluorescein angiography shows early hyperfluorescence of the white lesions. ERG shows a decreased a-wave, suggesting abnormal outer retinal dysfunction. The condition usually resolves spontaneously with good visual recovery.

224 In lamellar cataracts:

a the lens opacity is between the cortex and the embryonic nucleus

b progression of the cataract after birth is common

c there are usually linear opacities extending from the cataract into the clear peripheral cortex

d the insult leading to the cataract usually occurs in the first trimester

e abnormal maternal calcium metabolism is a cause.

225 The following are true about piggyback intraocular lens implant:

a it is usually carried out in patients with a refraction of more than 30D

b spherical aberrations are more common than using one single lens

c a larger incision is required during surgery

d the lens with higher power is usually placed anterior to the lens with lower power

e interlenticular opacification is a complication.

226 Periorbital haematoma is a feature of:

a basal skull fracture

b amyloidosis

c neuroblastoma

d haemophilia A

e sickle cell anaemia.

227 In a patient whose pupils do not react to light but constrict with accommodation, the following signs may be an associated finding:

a vermiform movement of the eye

b small irregular pupils

c presence of optic atrophy in both eyes

d presence of extensive pan-photocoagulation

e convergence-retraction nystagmus.

224

Lamellar or zonular cataract is a congenital cataract characterised by the presence of lens opacities between the cortex and the embryonic nucleus. Two additional features are the presence of an envelope, which is a thin opacity surrounding the main cataract, and the presence of riders, which are linear opacities extending from the cataract into the clear cortex. The insult is thought to occur in late pregnancy. Abnormal maternal calcium metabolism such as hypoparathyroidism is a known factor. The condition is usually static.

225

Piggyback intraocular lens implants involve the use of two or more intraocular lenses to achieve the required post-operative power following cataract surgery. It is used mainly in patients with intraocular lens power of 30D or more. It has the advantage of causing fewer spherical and chromatic aberrations. The implants may be foldable and therefore the incision does not have to be larger. Lenses with lower power are usually placed anterior to lenses with higher power to facilitate intraocular lens exchange should adjustment of the refractive power be required. Opacification between the implants is a complication.

226

Basal skull fracture can cause bilateral periorbital haematoma (racoon's sign). Amyloidosis may lead to formation of fragile blood vessels which may bleed spontaneously. Orbital metastasis of neuroblastoma is also associated with spontaneous haemorrhage. Haemophilia A results in an abnormal clotting profile but does not cause spontaneous bleeding and neither does sickle cell anaemia.

227

Vermiform movement of the eye occurs in Adie's pupil. Small irregular pupils are seen in tertiary neuro-syphilis. Optic atrophy may stop the pupils from responding to light but not to accommodation. Extensive pan-photocoagulation can cause damage to the long ciliary nerve and subsequent aberrant regeneration can give rise to light-near dissociation. Convergence-retraction nystagmus is a feature of Parinaud's syndrome which in turn is associated with light-near dissociation.

228 The following pairings are correct:

a   Gerstmann's syndrome – dominant parietal lobe

b   prosopagnosia – bilateral frontal lobe lesion

c   achromatopsia – bilateral occipital lobe lesion

d   akinetopsia – middle temporal gyrus lesion

e   Anton's syndrome – bilateral parietal lobe lesion.

229 In retinitis pigmentosa:

a   the X-linked type tends to have worse visual prognosis than the autosomal dominant type

b   electrophysiology typically shows a normal a-wave but abnormal b-wave

c   visual field shows ring scotoma best shown on Humphrey perimetry

d   the macula may have oedema which does not leak on fluorescein angiography

e   the sectorial type typically involves the inferior retina.

230 The following conditions are associated with deafness:

a   Bardet-Biedl's syndrome

b   Norrie's disease

c   Kearne-Sayre's syndrome

d   Cogan's interstitial keratitis

e   Leber's congenital amaurosis.

231 Kaposi's sarcoma:

a   is caused by human herpes virus type 8

b   arises from the endothelium

c   typically causes blockage of lymphatic drainage

d   is confined to the skin

e   can be treated with antiviral agents.

228

Gerstmann's syndrome results from a lesion in the dominant parietal lobe. It is characterised by acalculia, agraphia, finger agnosia and left-right confusion. Prosopagnosia is an inability to recognise familiar faces and usually results from bilateral occipitotemporal involvement. Achromatopsia is abnormal colour discrimination and can arise from bilateral parietal or occipital lobe abnormalities. Akinetopsia implies insensitivity to motion and can result from a lesion in the middle temporal gyrus. Anton's syndrome occurs in blind patients who deny they are blind. It is seen in bilateral occipital lesions.

229

Retinitis pigmentosa may be autosomal dominant, X-linked or autosomal recessive. The autosomal dominant type tends to have the best visual prognosis. ERG shows abnormal a- and b-waves with eventual obliteration of both. The ring scotoma involves the periphery and is best shown on Goldman visual field. Cystoid macular oedema may occur but fluorescein angiography may not reveal leakage. Oral acetazolamide may be helpful. Sectorial retinitis pigmentosa is a variant and usually involves the lower retina.

230

Other conditions associated with deafness include:

- Usher's syndrome
- mucopolysaccharidoses
- Alport's disease
- congenital syphilis
- congenital rubella
- Vogt-Koyanagi-Harada's syndrome.

231

Kaposi's sarcoma is most commonly seen in AIDS patients. It is caused by human herpes virus type 8. The tumour originates in the endothelium of either blood or lymphatic vessels. The tumour commonly invades the lymphatic system, causing lymphoedema. It can affect not only the skin but the conjunctiva and orbit. Antiviral agents do not appear to be effective. Excision, radiation and systemic chemotherapy with either vincristine or vinblastine are effective.

232 The cover test:

a gives the same information as the alternating cover test

b can detect abnormal retinal correspondence

c can detect eccentric fixation

d is the best test for tropia

e can be used to detect dissociated vertical deviation.

233 In pituitary apoplexy:

a severe sudden headache is the typical presentation

b decreased vision with ophthalmoplegia is common

c occurs mostly in malignant tumour

d urgent resection of the tumour with steroid cover is necessary

e hypopituitarism is common.

234 During repair of a rhegmatogenous retinal detachment, the following are true regarding drainage of subretinal fluid:

a drainage is indicated if there is significant vitreoretinal traction

b drainage should be performed as close to the retinal hole as possible

c it can help to localise the retinal hole

d it is useful for softening the eye

e drainage should be performed before buckling.

235 Regarding herpes virus infections:

a conjunctival swapping for Lipschutz bodies is found in herpes simplex viral infections

b Giemsa staining of epithelial cells helps in the diagnosis of herpes simplex viral infections

c fluorescent antibody staining techniques demonstrate intracellular herpetic inclusion bodies

d varicella zoster infection of the lids can be confirmed by staining for Henderson Patterson bodies

d Tzanck smear is useful for identifying herpes virus.

232

The cover test is used to detect tropia, whereas the alternating cover/uncover test detects both tropia and phoria. Abnormal retinal correspondence and eccentric fixation cannot be detected with a cover test. Dissociated vertical deviation shows an upward movement of the eye when it is covered.

234

The indications for drainage of subretinal fluid are: presence of a bullous retinal detachment which is making localisation of a retinal tear or hole difficult; long-standing retinal detachment with viscous subretinal fluid; and inferior retinal detachment. Drainage should be performed before buckling and away from the retina break, as the use of cryotherapy at the site of drainage may cause problems.

233

Pituitary apoplexy occurs as a result of sudden enlargement of a pituitary adenoma either due to haemorrhage or infarction. The tumour is usually benign. The resultant mass can expand into the cavernous sinus, causing compression of the cranial nerves. Altered consciousness with decreased vision and ophthalmoplegia are common. In the acute stage, resection of the tumour with steroid cover can be life-saving. Hypopituitarism is a common outcome with or without surgery.

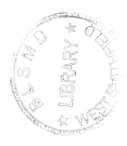

235

Lipschutz bodies, also called Cowdry type A inclusions, are seen in cells infected with herpes simplex or varicella zoster virus. They are best seen with the infected epithelial cells fixed in Bouin's solution and stained with Papanicolaou method. Giemsa stain shows up cells infected by the herpetic virus. The infected cells show multi-nucleation with balloon degeneration. Immunofluorescence can identify cells infected with herpes virus. Henderson Patterson bodies refer to eosinophilic cytoplasmic inclusion bodies seen in molluscum contagiosum. Tzanck smear involves scraping the base of a vesicle and inoculating it onto a microscopic slide. The syncytial giant cells which are characteristic of cells infected with the herpes virus can be demonstrated with Wright's or Giemsa stain.

236 Superior limbic keratoconjunctivitis:

a is associated with superior follicular tarsal conjunctivitis

b causes hypertrophy of the superior limbus

c is associated with filamentary keratitis

d can be diagnosed with impression cytology

e shows a favourable response with silver nitrate to the upper tarsal conjunctiva.

237 The ocular complications of bone marrow transplantation include:

a cataract

b keratoconjunctivitis sicca

c cotton wool spots

d cicatricial lagophthalmos

e corneal keratinisation.

238 Enlargement of the optic canal occurs in:

a carotid cavernous fistula

b fibrous dysplasia

c sphenoidal meningioma

d ophthalmic artery aneurysm

e optic nerve glioma.

239 Vitamin B_{12} deficiency:

a produces a decrease in central vision with relative sparing of peripheral vision

b does not affect colour vision

c may cause retinal haemorrhages

d causes temporal pallor of the optic nerve in long-standing cases

e is the actual cause of alcohol-tobacco amblyopia.

236

Superior limbic keratoconjunctivitis is a chronic condition involving the superior limbus and cornea and the superior tarsal conjunctiva. The changes in the tarsal conjunctiva are typically papillary. The limbus is often thickened. Although the diagnosis is usually made clinically, in doubtful cases, impression cytology of the superior bulbar conjunctiva can be useful and this usually shows nuclear pyknosis, loss of goblet cells and keratinisation. Treatment includes the use of silver nitrate to the upper tarsal conjunctiva, resection of the bulbar conjunctiva and the use of a large-diameter contact lens.

237

Following bone marrow transplantation some patients can develop graft-versus-host disease. In the chronic form, patients may develop cataract, ocular surface abnormalities such as keratoconjunctivitis sicca, corneal keratinisation and skin abnormalities such as cicatricial lagophthalmos. Rarely, cotton wool spots and haemorrhages have been observed.

238

A lesion of the optic nerve can cause enlargement of the optic canal and this is seen in optic nerve meningioma and glioma. Ophthalmic artery aneurysm also causes enlargement. Carotid cavernous fistula does not affect the canal size. Sphenoidal meningioma causes hyperostosis and may reduce the size of the canal.

239

Vitamin B_{12} deficiency may give rise to optic neuropathy. Colour vision is affected and the visual field may show central or centrocecal scotoma. The posterior pole typically shows flame-shaped and dot-blot retinal haemorrhages. Temporal pallor of the optic nerve is common. It is a cause of amblyopia in alcohol-tobacco amblyopia.

240 The following lesions may be responsible for a Horner's pupil that dilates with 0.1% adrenaline:

a   Pancoast's tumour

b   syringomyelia

c   post-thyroidectomy

d   internal carotid artery aneurysm

e   post-sympathectomy for Raynaud's phenomenon.

240

A normal pupil does not react to 0.1% adrenaline. However, in patients with post-ganglionic third-order lesions, denervation hypersensitivity develops, causing the pupil to dilate with 0.1% adrenaline. Pancoast's tumour causes a second-order lesion and syringomyelia causes a first-order lesion. Third-order lesions may occur in post-thyroidectomy patients, internal carotid artery aneurysms and post-sympathectomy.

Quick fix

- The following drops can be used to diagnose anisocoria: 4% cocaine, 1% pilocarpine, 0.1% pilocarpine, 1% hydroxyamphetamine and 0.1% adrenaline.

- A miotic pupil that does not dilate with 4% cocaine suggests Horner's syndrome.

- A miotic pupil caused by pre-ganglionic Horner's syndrome will dilate with 1% hydroxyamphetamine due to intact third-order neurones which release noradrenaline in response to 1% hydroxyamphetamine. A post-ganglionic Horner's pupil will not dilate with 1% hydroxyamphetamine.

- A miotic pupil caused by post-ganglionic Horner's syndrome will dilate with 0.1% adrenaline due to denervation hypersensitivity. A pre-ganglionic Horner's pupil will not dilate with 0.1% adrenaline.

- A mydriatic pupil that does not constrict with 1% pilocarpine suggests pharmacological mydriasis (for example, atropine).

- A mydriatic pupil that constricts with 0.1% pilocarpine suggests Adie's pupil due to denervation hypersensitivity.

Fact Finder

Fact Finder

Fact Finder

Fact Finder

Fact Finder

Fact Finder